HEALING
YOUR RELATIONSHIP
WITH FOOD

The Ayurveda Answer

MEENA PURI

This wonderful work by Ms. Meena Puri is filled with practical tools and profound wisdom that will allow you to cut through all the confusion of fad diets and change how you view food and your life forever! Ms. Puri's vision for a healthier tomorrow is clearly heartfelt and will inspire us all to take an active role in creating healthier communities. What's more, her book is a powerful reminder to all health practitioners to open our minds to that which is most important: the patients who trust us to guide them to healing. Food is medicine, and Ms. Puri includes delicious recipes in this beautiful book that will allow you to fill your kitchen with healing foods designed to turn you into your own Health Hero!

I have a profound respect for Eastern Medicine, especially when it's combined with the marvels of modern Western Medicine, and this book, filled with compelling stories, shows how Eastern concepts of going to the root of the disease can enhance the future of Western medical practice. The principles elucidated in this work will help pave the way for a healing journey that will allow you to derive ever more enjoyment than ever before from your life. It's truly a powerful addition to your bookshelf!

Dr. Partha Nandi
Creator and host of The Dr. Nandi Show

We usually think of food as nourishing us with vitamins and minerals and providing energy to us. Meena Puri goes under that science to the essential Consciousness that is available through our right relationship with food. She blends this delicious depth with very practical tips on what and how to eat for healthful living. Her book will nourish your body and your soul.

Rhonda Egidio, Ph.D.
Professor of Education Michigan State University, Ayurveda Practitioner.

Meena Puri's conscious approach to food and relationship with food provides an outline for a systematic approach to various silent, intricate features of health and wellness. This book offers not only cooking recipes, but also provides vast knowledge of Ayurvedic approach to food and nutrition. As I teach and conduct various Ayurvedic Food and Nutrition Consultant certification trainings, Meena Puri's book will be a valuable resource in helping students and practitioners understand various concepts of Ayurvedic nutrition. Her book is also highly beneficial and recommended for registered dieticians and anyone seeking to understand Ayurvedic nutrition.

Dr. Shekhar Annambhotla, President,
Association of Ayurvedic Professionals of North America (AAPNA), Inc. USA.

Even if you think you know every thing about food, this book is a must read. Bringing balance in our body and our life is something we face daily and to think we can do that with the foods we consume is quite a discovery. Much more than a diet or a recipe book, the wisdom offered here will help you bring balance and healing in your kitchen and… your life. Obsessed with counting calories, we overlook the most important ingredient in our nutrition, that is the energy it holds and imparts to our body and our mind and how it affects our Consciousness. The wisdom offered here, where Ayurveda meets Western lifestyle, is profound for preventing disease and for healing.

The added bonus is the captivating prose that will invite you into the book and will ring true for you. It is a CLASSIC, to be read, reread, shared and gifted. Every paragraph is an aha moment.

Susan Niedzielski B.S. M.A.,
Educator, Yoga Teacher, Ayurveda Practitioner

ISBN: 978-1-7328793-0-0

Published by Ayurvedic Healing Center LLC

Photos by Simone Kitschke
Cover Design by Trevor Stooke
Book Design by Janet Rouss

The Information in this book is based on Ayurvedic Principles that have been practiced for thousands of years. I encourage you to use the information to promote self healing. It is not intended, however, to replace professional medical care or treatment. For any medical conditions, always consult a licensed health care professional.

A tribute to my father.

If only I had your wisdom.

The art of healing comes from nature,
not from the physician. Therefore the physician
must start from nature, with an open mind.

Phillipus Aureolus Paracelsus

CONTENTS

Foreword xv

Preface xvii

How this book is organized .xxiii

Section I   Our Challenges 1

Chapter 1 Guilt and Shame 3

Chapter 2 Emotional Hunger 9

Chapter 3 Our Disconnection from Food. 23

Chapter 4 Overconsumption and Addiction 37

Chapter 5 Lack of Personal Responsibility 45

Section II   Ayurveda Offers Solutions 51

Chapter 6 Ayurveda Fills the Gap 53

Chapter 7 Consciousness and its Role in Healing 65

Chapter 8 The Bigger Context 69

Chapter 9 Our Connection with Creation 73

Chapter 10 Energy, Quality, and Balance 101

Chapter 11 Digestibility. 107

Chapter 12 What Makes Food Ayurvedic? 115

CONTENTS

Section III   **Healing: A Collective Concept**. 123

Chapter 13 It Takes a Village. 125

Chapter 14 I Dream of a Different World 129

Chapter 15 Food is Our Medicine. .135

Section IV   **Recipes: Let the Healing Begin in Your Kitchen**. . .141

Chapter 16 Stocking Your Ayurvedic Pantry 143

Chapter 17 Be Your Own Master Chef 147

Chapter 18 Notes About the Recipes 149

Chapter 19 Recipes 153

More About the Author 201

Bibliography. 202

End notes 203

ACKNOWLEDGEMENTS AND GRATITUDE

Years ago, I volunteered to host a Yoga Fundraiser to help a student serve kids in an underdeveloped community in Peru. We had a great turnout and I was able to fit 22 students into my small home studio. We used every inch of the space in the studio and I managed to teach Yoga while I was practically plastered to the wall.

The highlight of the event was the Indian lunch I had prepared. Plans to eat outside were undermined by an unusually strong wind, so at meal-time I lined my living room and kitchen with tables and chairs. It turned out to be a memorable experience for all, and, most importantly, we raised over $700. This money went a long way to help the kids in Peru.

It was at this event that many participants suggested I teach a cooking class, as they had really enjoyed the lunch. Of course, I laughed it off as I had never followed a recipe or measured anything while cooking. I did it all instinctively and by feel. In order to teach, I would have to write out the exact recipes and that felt like a jarring idea; it felt like work I didn't want to do.

The suggestions were sincere and persistent, however. I mentioned the idea to my friend, Alison, who not only gave me encouragement, but also transcribed a recipe while I talked it out. This led to me teaching a class on the secrets of Indian Cooking in a middle school's skills room, to about 15 people. They not only thoroughly enjoyed the dishes we had prepared, but really appreciated learning all about the spices; they loved being able to add new dishes to their repertoire.

What followed were more cooking classes and after I graduated from Ayurveda School, I started to teach an Ayurvedic nutrition and cooking program right out of my kitchen. I fielded constant requests for a cookbook. That fundraiser meal really was the starting point for this book, which started out as a way to share the recipes but ended with a lot more than that. I've learned that anything can turn into the first step towards an unknown future, or even to a goal that we may have never imagined. I am grateful to all those who encouraged me and suggested I write this book. I am especially grateful to my friend, Alison, who transferred that one recipe from my head to paper and made me realize that writing a recipe down was not all that difficult after all.

With the yoga studio housed right below my kitchen, my students often say things like, "It smells so good. What are you cooking? You should do a book!" Thank you for your kind and encouraging comments, your trust and, moreover, for appreciating the meals that I prepare at our meditation retreats and special events.

I have thoroughly enjoyed cooking the recipes that you will find in this book, particularly because of my friend and photographer, Simone Kitschke. Without her, this book would not be possible. We had many sessions of cooking, taking pictures, eating and repeating this pattern, and we had a blast. My Indian passion and her German discipline could not have been a better match, and I can say that we were in the "zone" every session. Things flowed and came together seamlessly. We also got immediate feedback on the recipes from her husband, our "lab rat," and Simone called me a mad scientist better fitted for an entertainment show than a cooking show. Thank you, Simone! I wonder what we will do next?

Many thanks to my editor Susan Crossman, not only for her support of my ideas and passion but for questioning me enough to pull a book out of me and for being there every time I needed a sounding board. There are so many others who have contributed to this book through their encouragement, feedback, support and their trust in me. Amongst those are my leaf sisters and colleagues Rhonda Egidio and Sue Niedzielski. I will always remember my book being read to me by you both. And thanks to my business coach, Sherri Richards, who told me it will only take me a month to write a book; it didn't but you did inspire me. I am grateful for Dr. Shekhar Annambhotla for his continuous support in whatever I do. I am grateful for my dear client, Chuck Hammond, for trusting in my work and offering many valuable suggestions and quotes for the book. I am always grateful for my family and my friends for believing in me and always cheering me on.

Last but not least, I am grateful for all of my teachers, including the ones who came in the guise of tough clients and students. You have taught me more than you will know. But in particular, I want to offer my deepest gratitude to the one and only Dr. Paul Dugliss, my teacher and mentor, who opened the world of Ayurveda and healing to me in the most authentic, compassionate and complete way possible. With such a strong foundation, I can only rise and I am forever grateful for him.

I dedicate this book to all of my students and clients. It is my sincere hope that through my thoughts, stories and the handful of recipes I have included here, you can become self-reliant and confident enough to not only take care of your basic need for food, but to gain a much broader understanding of what it means to be "healthy." I hope you enjoy following these recipes as much as I have enjoyed putting them together for this book, and that they serve you well for years to come.

To Your Happy Health,

Meena Puri
Milford, MI October 2018

FOREWORD

You are in for a pleasant surprise with this book. It is so much more than a cookbook or even an introduction to Ayurvedic Nutrition. What Meena has done is offer a wonderful exploration of eating and enjoying food that integrates the profound insights of the East with the modern world of the West. She is a unique presenter — highly qualified to bridge East and West, and she does this in a way that is full of authenticity and practicality.

What you will learn about in this book is that which is most near and dear to you. Meena gives a treasure trove of wisdom and knowledge about you — about your inner psychology and about how your body works. This is the inner secret of Ayurveda and these secrets are made available through her personal experience and her years of practice applying the art and science of Ayurvedic nutrition with her clients. She cuts through all the confusion and the allure of fad diets and all of the conditioning that we have had since childhood around eating. She restores the most fundamental truth of life — that food is to be enjoyed. And she shows how this can be done in a way that is simple and healthy.

This book goes way beyond the common exposition of Ayurvedic Nutrition as knowing the doshic quality of a food and thus what body type it might be good for. It is one thing to look up that knowledge. It is quite another thing to be able to integrate Ayurvedic principles around digestion and healthy diet into our modern culture. This is Meena's forte.

So, while you may be attracted to this book by its colorful and appealing photos, know that you are in for a real treat — an exploration of how to return to simplicity and common sense when it comes to eating that frees us to be able to enjoy and digest and utilize food as never before.

Those who have been blessed to have experienced Meena's cooking know that this book is full of wonder. If you haven't had that pleasure, then you may feel her laughter and her caring spirit coming through the words and recipes you are about to experience.

Take these gifts and know that this book represents the best combination of higher wisdom and practical knowledge presented in a down-to-Earth manner.

Enjoy!

Paul Dugliss, M.D.
Ayurveda Specialist and Practitioner of Traditional Chinese Medicine
Academic Dean and Director of New World Ayurveda
Author of Enlightened Nutrition, Ayurveda - the Power to Heal, Capturing the Bliss, Ayurveda and the Yoga of Emotions, Living Beyond Your Wildest Dreams, Think with the Heart, Love with the Mind, Patanjali in the Light

PREFACE

I grew up in a small town in India where there were no restaurants. I never saw food in a can, or a freezer, and it rarely came in a package. We did not own a fridge for the longest time. In fact, in our neighborhood, only one family had a fridge. We often went to their house for ice with which to make lemonade in the summers. When we did finally get a fridge, it was treated like a prized possession and my mom put it in a corner of our living room with some decorations on top. The fridge was a gift from my brother, who lived in Canada. He bought it for us one day when he came home to visit. There was to be no more running to the neighbor's house for ice for us and, as a bonus, we started to make mango ice-cream. No fruits or vegetables ever went into the fridge. We actually did not know what to use it for.

In contrast, we had four kitchens. Yes, we did! Anytime there was an addition made to the house, my mom made sure to put a kitchen in it. In those days kitchens were very basic and small. I don't remember ever seeing an electronic gadget in one, but there would be a portable pantry, a few open shelves for dishes, maybe a small cabinet with some food in clay and tin jars inside, perhaps some pickles, a wooden box for spices and some other dried food. One of our kitchens was on a rooftop, right outside the indoor kitchen. The outdoor kitchen included a stove made out of clay. It had an opening in it through which we would put wood and cow dung patties for fire. We adjusted the heat by either pulling the wood out or putting more in. The indoor stoves were made of clay and metal, and we used coal for fire. No push of a button and minor adjustment of a dial to control the heat, not to mention the fact that on damp days, it took some doing to start the fire; there was also smoke to deal with. We cooked our food while sitting down on a stool and we sat on the kitchen floor to eat it hot and fresh. Food has never tasted as good to me since then. It was Simple Goodness!

Food was made fresh at meal times and rarely were there leftovers. Sometimes we ate together and many times one person cooked while the others ate. Baking was something we did not do, as ovens were uncommon. Every now and then, we would outsource the baking of cookies to someone who did have an oven. We would give him the ingredients—flour, butter and sugar—and, in return, we would get a tin full of cookies. My mom or sisters made fresh snacks whenever the desire struck. So, overeating was never really an issue. Being the youngest, I cooked the least and did most of the running around, fetching this or that. But during summer holidays, I had to have a turn cooking. I remember playing with dough and cutting it with round sharp bowls to make a perfectly round chapati, which is Indian flat bread. Noticing that I played more than I cooked and was too slow, my sister generally dismissed me. Today it is hard to imagine that I was ever slow at anything, but that is the family rumor.

Food nourished us on many levels. It was never used as a reward, nor as a punishment; there was never any talk of eating too much or eating too little. We ate when we were hungry and forgot about it the rest of the time. My dad, being a doctor, was very healthy and did not allow anything of poor quality into the house. We had an abundance of seasonal fresh fruit and vegetables. Being a large family of eleven kids, food disappeared quickly. Sometimes, one of us would take someone else's portion of that special snack that a guest had brought, or even eat it all, making my mom wonder what had happened to it. I don't remember feeling any guilt about food. Ever!

Using written recipes was unheard of. Knowledge and information about food was shared verbally and I learned to cook mostly just by being around food. The kitchen was the purest place in our home, kind of like a temple. Shoes were not allowed inside it, and it was cleaned after every meal. There were no dirty dishes lying around. And food was offered to The Gods on special occasions. It seemed like there was a special occasion every day. Every morning, the kitchen floor was washed, the soot that had accumulated from cooking the previous meal was cleaned out, and the clay stove was freshened with new clay. My mom would say that God does not enter a house with a dirty kitchen.

We had no TV in those days. When we ate, that's all we did. There were no distractions to distort the experience! There were fewer opportunities to overeat, as the amount of food prepared was tailored to the number of people in the house. With a large family, our concern was more about whether everybody would get enough to eat, rather than whether someone might overeat or whether there might be leftovers. We did not indulge in much conversation while eating. We simply ate! Imagine that! That naturally made us mindful of eating and experiencing what it was like to feel full and satisfied. We developed an internal reference as to how much to eat. Chapati was made fresh at each meal and served hot off the grill as soon as it was ready. When we were full, we simply did not take any more food. We were never told to finish what was on our plate, as not all of the meal was served to us at once. It is interesting how the "clean plate club" and the idea of "overeating" in our society are concepts that developed as our eating, cooking and lifestyles changed. With so much struggle around overeating in our society, generally, I wonder if cooking food fresh for each meal might be the ideal solution for us all.

I had never heard of processed food while I was growing up. I left India in my teen years to study in Toronto. While going to school in Toronto, it never occurred to me to look at the list of ingredients in the food I bought. The idea that there would be something else in my food *other* than food was foreign to me. So, I happily ate those Kraft cheese singles thinking that they were made only of cheese.

I am certain my story speaks to many of us. Today, some 35 years on, we have a plethora of food plans, diets, guilt-free and zero-calorie foods, calorie-logging programs and apps, and an epidemic of illnesses never heard of before. Coincidence? I think not! Moreover, the information overflow and limitless choices we face around food keep us wondering and worrying whether we've got it all, whether we really know everything there is to know. Regardless of how hard we try to wrap our heads around food, we keep missing the mark.

How did we get here? On one hand, we are fortunate to have an abundance and variety of foods, yet, on the other hand we are anxious and worried and we struggle to eat healthily. Is it the information overflow? Is it the ease with which we can obtain so much food? Is it our sedentary, stressful and push-button lifestyle?

In a world of quick and easy recipes, power foods and shakes, groceries delivered to our doorsteps and meals prepared and dropped off for us, we are saving a lot of time, yet the biggest dilemma of our times is our perceived lack of time. With the most nutrient-dense foods possible available to us, the worry about nutritional deficiencies remains. Hand-in-hand with that is fear, anxiety and confusion. I have often wondered if having too many options isn't part of the problem. Those who love the "options" world—and don't get me wrong, I do too—may frown upon this idea. I am certain this is a problem, although I'm not sure what the solution is. But it makes me want to say, "Wait a minute!" When a so-called solution (endless information) comes with another set of problems (confusion and anxiety), then perhaps we are better off with the original problem. Either way, going back to the basics may be the way to solve it.

Knowing less and applying what we already know may be what's needed, instead of figuring our way out of this mess with another miracle food, more recipes, or another diet plan. From the beginning of time, food was meant to sustain, to nourish, to heal, to connect and to celebrate life. Perhaps much of the food-related illnesses we are suffering as a society are the result of not just the "bad food" but rather from the lack of emotional and psychological nourishment we receive. Is there something we are bypassing when we don't chop, cut, stir and prepare our own meals? Our body is made up of a complex set of processes that occur step by step. Can we really outsmart our bodies and skip steps just for the sake of convenience and time?

The process of chopping, cutting, mixing and stirring is an understated yet important part of our digestive system. It inspires the senses and starts the digestive process. As we smell the food, we begin to salivate, which wakes up our digestion in anticipation of a delicious meal. Moreover, the aromas, different textures, and colors wake up our subtle senses and make our entire body receptive of the nourishment it is about to receive.

The subtle part of our being is the most powerful part that drives the intelligent functioning of our internal organs and systems. The digestive process allows us to not just enjoy the foods we are eating, but also to be nourished by what we eat. When food goes straight from the box to the mouth, we have to ask if our body is truly ready to digest, to process, and to make use of this food as fuel for our soul, our psyche and our physical body? I wonder if we don't take a hit on more than just the physical level every time we end up in front of the window of a fast food restaurant, or grab that frozen meal.

In our busy lives, we have begun to value convenience, but I wonder if we have forsaken joy and happiness for the sake of convenience. Quality and fullness of life are a result of the experiences we have. It might be constructive to ask what adds value to our lives and what diminishes it.

Nothing gets more in the way of our aspirations, our goals and our ability to live a purposeful life than ill health, and nothing can stop us from living our rich and meaningful life when we are healthy from the inside out. Food and nutrition represent one of the big ways that we can all create real health. Food is a metaphor for life; if we can heal our relationship with food, we can heal our life.

If we continue to search for the "perfect" food or diet out there, we have bought into the belief that someone else has the power to change our health. It is this belief that we need to shift. We must take the reins of our health into our own hands.

What's out there is *information*, but to transform our health what we need is *wisdom*. That source of wisdom is within each one of us. All that's needed is our willingness to try to access it!

I am convinced that the solution to our food-related problems lies in returning to basics, in simplifying nutrition, and in building a healthier relationship with our food and food sources. Most importantly, it lies in our willingness to use our common sense and ask the bigger questions when it comes to our struggles with food. I am certain that when we view food as our ally in creating long-lasting health and healing, we may be taking the single most important step in healing our relationship with food, regardless of what background, beliefs and associations we may have. I believe that food can be the source of health and healing. And, when viewed as such, it can be our most valuable resource in dealing with stress.

Food is life-giving and it is a celebration of life. May we cook together, eat together, laugh, rejoice and share stories over good food. May no one go hungry! May this simple need and pleasure be bestowed upon all human beings! May there be enough in our pantry, our fridge and our kitchen and may the kettle be always on. May our doors and, most importantly, our hearts, always be open to share this blessing with all!

HOW THIS BOOK IS ORGANIZED

This book is organized into four sections. Each new concept or thought is a new chapter. Where appropriate, the chapters end with a reflective statement or an action step to help you process the material a little more profoundly. Client and personal stories are included for teaching purposes and they are italicized. The client names are changed to maintain confidentiality and only what is needed for teaching purposes is shared.

Here is a little tour of each section:

SECTION I - OUR CHALLENGES

These are the top five challenges that I have encountered in my practice. Understanding the source of these challenges and how they affect our relationship with food have allowed me to address the problems that I see in people's lives. Everyone's challenges are unique and yours may not fit perfectly into any one category that I have listed. Reading through what I have presented may provoke thought, however, and help clarify for you where your difficulties lie.

There are five chapters in Section I. The first chapter talks about guilt and shame and how that gets in the way of having enjoyable experiences with food. The second chapter talks about emotional hunger which, until addressed and satisfied, will continue to hinder any progress we make in our healing. The third chapter talks about the disconnect we have with food and its source, and our body's innate intelligence when it comes to healing. Medicine and food are not separate. This chapter also talks about the protein and dairy concern and a better way to enjoy smoothies. The fourth chapter is about overconsumption and addiction. Finally, the fifth chapter points to the need to take personal responsibility in creating the health we want. Each chapter also provides some tools and techniques that you can begin to use right away. However, the ultimate solution is in our deep connection with Source and that is the subject matter of the next section.

SECTION II - AYURVEDA OFFERS SOLUTIONS

The ancient wisdom and science of Ayurveda offers the ultimate solutions to our modern day challenges. The first chapter introduces Ayurveda and how it fills the gap in our health and healing. This chapter outlines the five major concepts that we can look at to get a broader and more comprehensive view of food and nutrition. The five concepts are: Consciousness and how it heals, the need for a bigger context, our connection with Creation, energy, quality and balance, and, finally, digestibility, a process that is often missed in all the hype around food and nutrition. The five-element theory and its relationship to food, to our constitution, to seasons, to cycles of day, and different tastes are discussed in one of the chapters in this section. You will also find a quiz that you can fill out to understand your own constitution and imbalance. Digestion is discussed in detail in one of the chapters and it outlines many things you can do today to improve your digestion. Understanding balance and its role in healing is also discussed in this section. The last chapter of this section talks about what makes food Ayurvedic and what creates toxins (Ama). At the end of this section, I hope that you will have a general understanding of Ayurveda and come away with some practical tools on how to view food so you can bring balance into your eating and your kitchen. I have kept this section as general and as non-technical as I possibly can. What's most important is that it broadens your understanding and gets you to think about food in a whole new way. It is that type of thinking that is needed in order for us to see food as the medicine that it truly is.

SECTION III - HEALING: A COLLECTIVE CONCEPT

The point of this section is to go beyond our problems and solutions. We don't heal in isolation and we can't pretend that elements in the external world, such as food corporations and pharmaceuticals, don't play a role. As much as we are independent, we are also interdependent. We affect others and are affected by them. Although all we can do is create a change within ourselves, it is good to be aware of the external influences and norms that can potentially undermine our efforts. Paying attention, waking up and taking a strong stand by changing our actions are all necessary. What would we do if we weren't so vested in our illnesses and diagnoses? We must rise above our problems and connect with our deepest desires and aspirations. Healing comes from exactly that. This is the shortest section of the book, with only three chapters in it. Powerful concepts don't need to be many, only a few will do. The first chapter talks about how healing must be a collective concept for a healthier nation and how we, as individuals, can shift our mind to create a village of healing. The second chapter talks about what our world could be like if the medical and the healing world were not divided, and it expands our definition of health to more than a mere lack of physical symptoms. The third chapter is about creating a healing mindset, and looks at how believing in healing can lead us to heal our relationship with food.

SECTION IV - RECIPES: LET THE HEALING BEGIN IN YOUR KITCHEN

Along with recipes, you will see some tips on how to stock your pantry and how to feel comfortable in your kitchen, even if cooking is something new for you. I've included about 40 recipes and some of them are for foods you may have never seen or heard of before. These are the recipes I know, and this is how I cook and eat. Pick a recipe that calls out to you and give it a try. This is by no means a cookbook. The handful of recipes I've included are to help you get started and get a flavor for Ayurvedic recipes. In the recipe and food world, I believe less is more. With an expanded understanding of food and some basic skills, we can create our own recipes, and I urge you to do just that. I hope you enjoy the recipes and that they serve as a basis for you to expand your repertoire and broaden your horizon.

In working with clients in my clinical practice, I've realized two things. First, that in trying to keep up with the newest miracle food or diet, people are often missing out on enjoying their food. And, second, that the overflow of information about food that people are facing is actually getting in the way of them being able to clearly understand food and nutrition. Part of my work with my clients is to teach them how to simplify cooking and nutrition: to think of nutrition in a bigger context and, using their own experience and intuition, to know what's working for them.

I believe today's overflow of food-related information has created room for simplicity; endless and often contradictory scientific research on food has given rise to the opportunity for people to trust their intuition and experience, and given them permission to fall back on common sense. I have intentionally kept this book non-scientific and I invite you to rely on what you already know. Keep things simple. Trust your own experience and intuition about what you enjoy, and what feels better for your body. **Remember, science is derived from experiences; experiences are not derived from science.** We can't wait for science to catch up to begin to use our own common sense and wisdom.

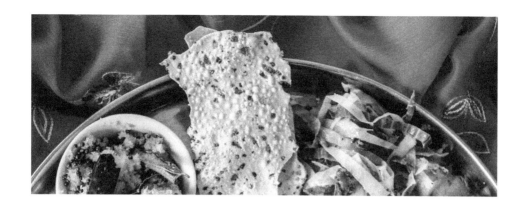

SECTION I

Our Challenges

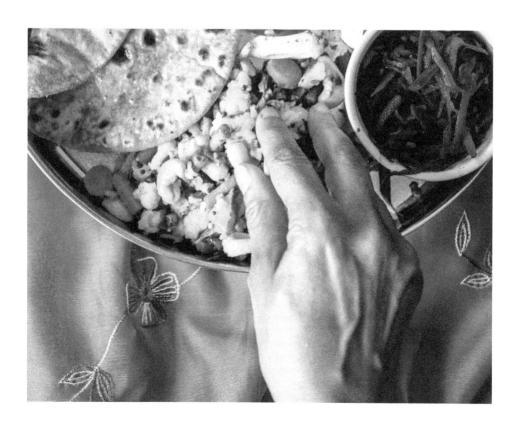

CHAPTER 1

Guilt and Shame

Emotional challenges are natural human challenges that teach us how to live in alignment with our truth with ease and presence. Our human life is about learning the lessons we are here to learn and eventually returning "Home." The more we learn, the more there is to learn. We never quite "get there" in one lifetime. We are always a work-in-progress. Our challenges are part and parcel of being human, and they simply serve as a catalyst along our journey to wholeness, which is our ultimate "Truth." This is neither heroic nor shameful. It just is! Welcome to life!

Accepting and embracing our challenges will go a long way in not only dealing with them when they strike, but also in opening up a world of possibilities, where we may view these difficulties as blessings that come to complete us! This mindset and understanding can serve as a template for how we live. Of course, we should seek solutions to our challenges and do everything we can to live happily. But when we accept our challenges as a means of enhancing our experience on this planet, we can approach them in a whole new way. The process becomes that of inquiry, discovery and intrigue, as opposed to desperation, fear and shame. We become empowered, not weakened. We want to approach our challenges from a place of power and never from a place of weakness. There is no longer a need to hide behind a problem because we understand it to be part and parcel of our human journey. When we don't hide a problem, we can solve it in the open, instead of dealing with it secretly and in less-than-desirable ways.

What does this have to do with food and eating?

Nothing! And everything!

If we are lucky, we have experienced the comfort, warmth and satisfaction that food can bring. These experiences represent our basic human needs and if they are missing in our life, we will naturally gravitate toward that which serves this need. A cup of tea on a cold wintery day can be just the thing to comfort us. A sweet treat as a way of self-love can sometimes do the trick, as well. Food is as much about spiritual and emotional nourishment as it is about nourishing our physical body. Fear of becoming over-reliant on food for our emotional nurturance can cause us to deny ourselves and feel guilty about deriving any pleasure from it.

On my son's 22nd birthday, I made him a chocolate chip cookie cake. I was generous with both butter and chocolate and made it extra decadent. Later he said, "Mom, it tasted so good, I honestly felt guilty about eating it." What is it about us humans that we feel guilty about getting any pleasure from food, I later thought?

Most, if not all of us, struggle with a lack of worthiness. Is it humility? Our ego? Are we just playing safe? I mean, we don't want to toot our own horn! What if we believed we were good enough but then later told that we weren't?! As I pondered this idea while writing this book, I realized that worthiness has nothing to do with our successes or failures: that would mean that each time we fail we are deemed unworthy, and that's simply not true! Worthiness is granted by that which created us. The Creator definitely thought we were all worthy, and created us all with an equal dosage of worthiness. Simply because we are born, we are worthy and good enough. Because we are on this planet, we are good enough. We are worthy of experiencing this human life, as difficult as it may sometimes be. We are worthy of learning the lessons set out for us and becoming whole. Worthiness is not the result of our accomplishments or lack thereof. Certainly, our challenges can make us question our worthiness and that's exactly when we should remember where we come from and who we truly are. We are good enough to enjoy the experiences we are here to experience, including decadent chocolate chip cookie cake.

INDULGING IS DESIRABLE

The guilt that keeps us from allowing ourselves the experience of pleasure equally pulls us into over-indulgence in trying to suppress it, and that keeps us stuck in a cycle of guilt and shame. However, indulging once in a while, or on special occasions, is desirable and allows us to truly experience enjoyment. In allowance, there is no guilt, only pleasure. And we may offer our gratitude for the experience. Instead of asking "Who am I to have such pleasure?" we might ask, "Who am I to not experience that pleasure?" As I heard from one of my teachers: when good things come into your life, simply say, "Thank you. May I have more please?" Because you are good enough!

Shame and guilt are the mental constructs of the mind to help us fit into the societal mold of what's right and wrong. These are merely our defense mechanisms, established to bridge the gap between what we want and what we think we should want. In this complex structure of feelings, the truth of what we actually feel and believe gets lost somewhere, or at least distorted, leaving most of us feeling insecure about what and how to eat; we chase the latest food craze, and coming up short every time. All this anxiety about food negatively affects our ability to digest it. We become hyper-sensitive to everything we eat. With every bite we take, we ingest a morsel of fear, guilt, shame and confusion right along with it. We believe we have no right to enjoy our food anymore, making that gap between what we want and what we should want bigger and bigger, and leaving food to fill that gap. Calling some foods "guilt-free" only emphasize the misplaced guilt we experience in eating and nourishing ourselves. The comfort we derive from food turns to guilt and shame if we don't resolve the deeper emotional challenges that are keeping us from living full, vibrant lives.

Dawn (one of my clients) brought her mother, Doris, to see me and, with her mother's consent Dawn stayed with her during the consultation. Doris was experiencing heat rash all over her arms and she attributed it to the hormone therapy she was undergoing. In trying to uncover the true cause of the problem, I asked for details of the food she was eating, as I always do, and nothing really pointed to what she was experiencing. Hormone therapy affects everyone differently and it can result in skin rash, but I wanted to rule out any other causative factors.

In the middle of the appointment, Doris asked to use the restroom and in her absence her daughter told me that her mother was a closet eater. Doris apparently ate a lot of salty chips when no one was looking. When Doris returned, I mentioned that in spite of how healthy her diet seemed to be, it was rather bland and lacked variety. I mentioned that when we don't have all the tastes and textures in our meals, we tend to seek them out through junk food, at which point Doris told me about her cravings for salty and crunchy things. She was overdoing it on the salt to compensate for the lack of it in her meals. This created more heat in her body, another contributing factor to her skin rash.

Doris thought that in order to stay healthy, she had to deny what she liked. That's often the case, as we believe that if it tastes good, it may not be too healthy for us. We can thank our marketing world for keeping us confused when it comes to food. "This tastes good, and it is even good for you," the marketing messages tell us, as if tasty and healthy are mutually exclusive. The truth is that we can choose many tasty foods that are also good for us.

WORK THROUGH THE PAIN

Fear can be debilitating. We lose our ability to navigate through emotional pain; perhaps we fear getting stuck in the pain and not being able to come out, even though that very pain is subconsciously ruling our lives and keeping us stuck in a pattern already! The quicker path to emotional liberation is to work through the pain. Unfortunately, as painful emotions surface, the fear of facing them makes us turn to food over and over again, always in the hope of eliminating these perceptively negative feelings. If food really could eliminate negative feelings, of course, we would eventually stop turning to it to try to satiate our emotional hunger. The only way out of the negative feelings is through them; we must allow them and feel them fully.

Allowing is a skill that we can all cultivate through practice. Seemingly difficult, the easiest thing to do is to feel what you feel! Surrender! Feel the fear! Feel bad! You may feel that your life is spinning out of control. Let it! Stay with it! Soon enough, you will feel tired or hungry or may need to go to the bathroom. Life goes on! The sun is still there, either shining or waiting behind the clouds. You are still here! The Earth did not shatter! You may feel awful, but you are OK.

Through feeling the pain, you will get to the other side of it, where there is peace.

When we work through the mind-directed emotions, we find only peace and love in our hearts. Fill yourself with that love by simply feeling it. Now you can spare food to simply nourish you, which is what it was meant to do!

The deeper beliefs that we are unlovable and unworthy can't be resolved with food, as we eventually discover. And what if we were viewing food as the temporary solution to a problem that had nothing to do with food? Now, on top of feeling unworthy, we begin to feel guilt and shame, since we know that what we are doing is not going to serve us, yet we can't stop. The more we suppress our feelings, the stronger they become. We get stuck in an insidious cycle, not only perpetuating our painful feelings, but embedding them deeper into our subconscious. Our basic human need to feel loved and worthy gets undermined when we use food to satisfy it. The brain becomes confused about whether to satisfy the physical hunger or the emotional hunger. The lines become blurry and we begin to play a game of "hide and seek" with food. What once was a pleasurable and satisfying experience becomes this phantom that we either run to or run from: controlling and logging every morsel that goes into our mouth or eating with reckless abandon, ignoring the physical symptoms of being full, yet remaining unsatisfied. How do we find that middle ground?

GUILT ABOUT WORLD HUNGER

Many of us feel guilty when we see world hunger or other forms of suffering in the world. Our problems may begin to seem very small and irrelevant by comparison. The mind thinks, "It could have been me, I have no right to have what I have when there is so much suffering in the world." The heart immediately connects us to others and feels their pain. Guilt may show that we care, but it does not take care of the problem we care about.

One of the hardest things I had to learn in my clinical practice was that there are no victims. The truth is, we are all here on our solo journeys, with different lessons to learn. The experiences we go through are what our soul must experience. This is one of the mysteries of life and we can't do much but surrender to it. We realize how little we know.

This does not mean we don't show compassion and extend a helping hand. But we can't do that by feeling guilty about the blessings we have in our life. We can be grateful for all that we have, and perhaps spare a prayer for those less fortunate than we are. We have the opportunity to replace guilt with humility, gratitude, prayer and compassion. Now we may be able to be of assistance.

WASTE NOT, WANT NOT?

"Finish the food on your plate, you can't waste it, especially when there is so much hunger in the world," might be words you have heard in the past. For many of us, they bring out guilt, which only results in overeating. The fact is that when we overeat, or feel we must clean our plate, we don't resolve world hunger, we simply overeat. This not only results in physical illness, but it also negatively affects our mental health, as we either consume guilt with our food or simply overuse or rationalize our overeating by chalking it up to the guilt we feel about world hunger. However, we might possibly help resolve world hunger by buying and cooking smaller quantities of food, and putting less food on our plates. We can donate the money we save to organizations that work to lessen world hunger, or we can donate meals to families in need; there are countless ways to make a difference. We don't make the world a better place by dimming our own light.

Nor can we help others by harming ourselves; we can only help them if we help ourselves first. When we experience our own blessings and allow joy into our lives, we uplift those around us and that helps in its own small way to lessen world suffering. Instead of perpetuating suffering, we become a source of inspiration. In order for compassion and love to flow effortlessly to others, our own hearts must be filled with it. Anything less than that keeps us emotionally hungry. Let's explore that in the next chapter.

Is there a trace of guilt and shame in your struggle with food?

Can you think of any examples of how that shows up for you?

CHAPTER 2

Emotional Hunger

Emotions are at the center of every aspect of our life; they can either propel us towards a particular outcome or take us away from it. When we love what we do, we do more of it, but when our hearts are not into something, we drag our feet and eventually stop doing it. Whatever it is we do, we do it because we get emotional satisfaction from it.

Eating is no exception. Emotions and food are directly linked. Our physical satisfaction or nourishment is not separate from our emotional satisfaction. Most of us look forward to eating and we enjoy food. We can't think on an empty stomach. A cup of chai on a cold winter day is such a comfort. Coffee in the morning makes many people happy. Food is at the very center of our existence, our lives. The kitchen is where the family gathers. Food is a celebration of life, our connectedness, and a way to share love.

Our first experience of love was when we were fed by our mothers. Eating imparted the feelings of satisfaction, love, happiness, warmth, nourishment and comfort. I often hear clients who need to make some serious nutritional changes say, "This is how my partner loves me, by cooking for me." "Perhaps they can love you a little less," I have laughingly responded.

It is no surprise that when love is missing in our lives, we turn to food.

How we relate to food is how we relate to ourselves. When we eat well and healthily, we feel good and confident about ourselves and in our ability to take care of ourselves in a positive way; similarly, when we overeat, eat too little or eat unhealthily, we feel bad about ourselves. In that sense, all eating is emotional, however food can't be the only source of our emotional fulfillment. The problem arises when we turn to food to stuff down our painful emotions, or use food to make up for what we lack in other areas of our lives.

It is important to note that while most emotional eating is linked to unpleasant feelings, it can also be triggered by positive emotions, such as rewarding oneself for achieving a goal or celebrating a holiday, or a special event. Using food from time to time as a pick-me-up, or to celebrate, is not a bad thing. We have all experienced emotional eating at least once in our lives, if not more often. It is only a problem when it becomes a pattern that we can't break.

HERE IS WHAT EMOTIONAL HUNGER MIGHT LOOK LIKE:

- Making room for desert, even when we are already full
- Diving into a pint of ice-cream when we feel down
- Opening the refrigerator when we feel upset, angry, lonely, stressed, exhausted or just bored
- Rewarding ourselves with food or punishing ourselves by not eating at all! (binging or starving)
- Feeling powerless or out of control around food
- Eating out of nervousness
- Constantly thinking about food and eating
- Turning to food when painful emotions surface

Everyone's story is different and unique to them. Nonetheless, our internal struggles show up in our eating habits. Regardless of our reasons, food only provides a temporary solution. Eating for reasons other than hunger not only causes health problems, but it also does not take our challenges away. It actually stuffs the emotions deeper into our subconscious, making them even stronger and leading to more emotional eating; this keeps us stuck in the pattern.

Emotional hunger can be just as powerful as physical hunger and it's easily mistaken as such until we pay attention. It is important to figure out ways to differentiate the two. Here are the top five clues that I have summarized from Harvard Medical School Special Health Report.[1]

1. Emotional hunger comes on suddenly. It hits you in an instant and feels overwhelming and urgent. Physical hunger, on the other hand, comes on more gradually. The urge to eat doesn't feel as dire or demand instant satisfaction (unless you haven't eaten for a very long time).

2. Emotional hunger craves specific comfort foods. When you're physically hungry, almost anything sounds good—including healthy stuff. But emotional hunger craves fatty foods or sugary snacks that provide an instant rush. You feel like you need chocolate or pizza, and nothing else will do.

3. Emotional hunger often leads to mindless eating. Before you know it, you've eaten a whole bag of chips or an entire pint of ice cream without really paying attention to the food or fully enjoying it. Once you start, you can't stop; you must finish the whole bag of cookies. In that sense, it looks like an addiction. Often my clients will say, "I did not even remember eating the whole bag." When you're eating in response to physical hunger, you're typically more aware of what you're doing.

4. Emotional hunger isn't satisfied once you're full. You keep wanting more and more, often eating until you're uncomfortably stuffed. Physical hunger, on the other hand, doesn't need to be stuffed. You feel satisfied when your stomach is full.

5. Emotional hunger isn't located in the stomach. Rather than a growling belly or a pang in your stomach, you feel your hunger as a craving you can't get out of your head. You're focused on specific textures, tastes, and smells.

One of the insidious things about any negative cycle is that it is self-promoting. Emotional eating leads to more emotional eating. How can we break this cycle? I am a firm believer in the idea that how we do one thing is how we do everything. The way we eat is inseparable from our core beliefs about ourselves, about the world, and about life in general. As we bring more fulfillment and more balance into our lives, food does not take center stage, it simply becomes a necessary and enjoyable way to nourish ourselves.

The goal is to lessen the effect emotions have on our eating habits. But first we must understand the extent of this effect. I'm going to share some tools that have proven to work in my clinical practice. Some of them are simple and easy, while others require a longer process. Begin with what you can do today and build upon that one tiny step at a time. Every plan that you turn into action strengthens you and magnifies your self-reliance. Do not come from a place of despair or hopelessness; come from a position of strength. Build on your strengths. What else in your life have you overcome? You can overcome this issue as well, and here are some tips to assist you with that:

1. BECOME MORE AWARE

This is always on the top of my list of resolving any challenge. If I can impart one thing to a client, it is this. Without this tool, we will always be hopping from one solution to the next, as they will all prove to be temporary. We can't become aware just because we want to. As discussed in the next section, awareness is borne out of a level, or a field, of Consciousness. Higher levels of Consciousness give rise to deeper awareness and insights. If we exist at a lower level of Consciousness, we may be aware of what is on that particular level, but not necessarily what's really going on at the deep subconscious levels of our being. Please note that your level of Consciousness is not a measure of how wonderful a person you are; it simply relates to the level of insight that you may have about your life and the world, thus affecting the quality of your life in a way that is not conventionally considered. (A conventional quality of life may mean you are focused on material things and your status; your level of Consciousness is about the quality of your thinking and the depth of your understanding.)

Meditation is an ideal way to make conscious what is in the subconscious, and we'll talk more about that later. Moreover, it is a much-needed antidote to stress and anxiety, side effects of our modern lives. This is how we connect with our true nature or true Self. A meditation practice strengthens our connection with that part of ourselves that is beyond our body and mind, raising our level of awareness. Changes stick if they are internally driven rather than externally imposed. That's why developing awareness will have a much bigger impact on your life than your willpower.

Another simple way to raise your awareness is to journal what you are eating and how you are feeling. Let's call it a food and mood journal. Every time you overeat or feel compelled to reach for that ice cream or cookie, take a moment to figure out what triggered the urge to do that. If you backtrack, you'll usually find an unsettling event that kicked off the emotional eating cycle. Write this all down in your food and mood journal: what happened to upset you, how you felt before you ate, what you ate (or wanted to eat), what you felt as you were eating, and how you felt afterward.

If there is a pattern here, you'll see it emerge over time,. Maybe you always end up gorging yourself after spending time with a friend who is very critical. Or perhaps you stress eat after a phone call from a certain someone, or at family gatherings. This type of work will reveal the connection of your emotions to your eating habits.

2.   TUNE INTO YOUR CHILDHOOD BELIEFS

Were you always asked to finish all the food on your plate? Was food in abundance or barely enough? Were you rewarded for good behavior with ice-cream or pizza? Were you sent to bed hungry as a punishment? Or given cookies when you were feeling sad? Perhaps some of your eating is driven by nostalgia, i.e. eating certain foods makes you feel connected to your tribe and to your past. To what extent are these beliefs shaping your beliefs about food today? Are these beliefs still in alignment with who you are now? Are they serving you? If not, it is wise to cut the cord with them. (Visualize a cord between you and the belief and, using imaginary scissors, cut that cord). Remember, you are cutting the cord connecting you with those beliefs, not the people who "gave" them to you. What new beliefs can you put in place to build a new foundation for yourself?

Our beliefs and habits need periodic review and renewal. Just as we change our wardrobe or the color of paint in our homes, so should we upgrade our beliefs every now and then, too. Certain beliefs need changing to continuously align with our higher purpose and values.

Another point that is worth making is that regardless of how we were raised, ultimately our life is our own responsibility. Our caregivers and parents do what they know to do. The point of visiting our childhood is to gain insight into the belief patterns that may be at play in our adult life, it is not to blame all of our challenges on our upbringing, as the ultimate responsibility rests with each one of us.

Holding on to beliefs that no longer serve us can make us sick on all levels. The disease manifestation is a process that started a long time ago in our subconscious mind and eventually expressed itself in our body as a full-blown physical symptom. We don't see the disease in the making and we mistakenly believe it to be only physical; we thus limit treatment to just the physical aspect of who we are. Modern medicine does that quite well, hopping from symptom to symptom, bandaging them all up but rarely getting to the root cause. I have yet to meet a client whose physical symptoms did not have a big psychological component. The disease is the unresolved story or conflict that resulted from holding on to old beliefs that you know are no longer true but can't seem to release. Masking the symptoms confuses our physiology and mentally debilitates us in very subtle, yet powerful, ways. We can't afford to not pay attention to that!

3. DEVELOP YOUR EMOTIONAL INTELLIGENCE

That's a big phrase! However, it just means that we are willing to look at our emotions to gain more insight into who we are and what we need. Our feelings are a window into our inner world. They help us understand and discover our deepest desires and fears, our frustrations, and the things that will make us happy. Is food filling in for what's otherwise lacking in your life? How else can you fulfill your emotions other than through food?

Feeling painful emotions isn't fun. You may fear being overwhelmed by them and not know how to find your way back through them. But having them control your life is far worse. And the truth is that when we don't obsess over or suppress our emotions, even the most painful and difficult ones subside relatively quickly and lose their power to control our attention. Learning to surrender to our emotions is a skill that we can easily master by practice. Here is a meditation on allowing. Read it to understand it and then give it a try.

Meditation on Allowing

Find a comfortable place to sit or lie down. Close your eyes and get settled in your body. Pay attention to your breath and let it become slow and relaxed. What's most painful in your life right now? Invite that in, recalling the details of the situation. Allow yourself to feel all the emotions that are associated with it: pain, anger, frustration or whatever they may be. Imagine that the whole scenario or the experience that generated those emotions is happening right now. Let this experience fill your entire body from head to toe. Stay with this and keep inviting the feelings in; allow them to fill your entire being. How intense are these emotions? Can you name them? Where in your body are you feeling them the most? Are they in one particular place or are you feeling them all over? Or perhaps you can't quite tell? Keep feeling them with a gentle attention on your breath. Perhaps you are beginning to cry? It is okay. Continue and simply feel what you feel. Notice if there is any change in how you are feeling. Are you still feeling as intense as when you started? If so, don't rush to change how you feel. Allow it to be as it is! Just be as you are. Has anything changed? Does it feel okay for you to open your eyes? If not, continue to sit, allow yourself to feel what you feel and open your eyes when it feels okay to open them.

By allowing the painful emotions, you worked through them and here you are! Still okay! You may no longer be gripped by those emotions once you are not afraid of feeling them. You may feel a sense of surrender, a gentle letting go, and perhaps some sadness. What typically happens in this meditation is that the emotions transform from fear to sadness and it is the sadness that we were so afraid to feel. The allowance is what makes our sorrows sweet, causes the tears to flow and opens our heart to love. Ultimately, love is all we wanted in the first place, and now it is here, right in our hearts.

In a culture that is fixated on controlling everything, allowing may be a foreign concept. I have come to realize that there is very little that we can actually control and the only response is to simply allow events to unfold. Feelings can't be purposefully "fixed," they can only be allowed and felt. Allowing "fixes" them.

Life can certainly be downright hard at times, but we make matters worse for ourselves when we believe life should be anything other than what it is! As painful as it is to feel deeply, controlling how we "should" feel would make it far worse. We must surrender to life in all its glory in order to come alive fully. This is how we show up for our life and for ourselves. Like one of my teachers from long ago said, "I never promised you a rose garden," to which my answer used to be, "Well, someone should!" And that someone turned out to be only me. Darn! And there is no rose garden, only the rose colored glasses—my perception.

4. TAKE TIME TO EAT

Treat eating as an activity like any other activity that you make time for. Sit down and eat in a settled and peaceful environment. Chew your food well and take time to savor your food. And don't rush away right after eating. Offer gratitude for the food you are to consume and all that took place for it to be on your plate. Eating is a sacred act that not only nourishes us on a physical level, but also on a psychological level. It's important to give yourself permission to eat what you enjoy at mealtimes. I have never told my clients to eat something because it is good for them unless they like it because happiness is the most important ingredient in improving your digestion.

We are a culture that is big on snacking, yet snacking can result in overeating: it doesn't allow you to feel completely satisfied like you would be if you sat down and had a meal. We remain physically and emotionally hungry. **When we don't take the time to eat, we end up eating all the time.** Skipping meals is another big trend in our society, as if it is a badge of importance or busyness. Anytime we skip a meal, we end up more than making up for it at the next meal. The truth is that when we sit down and eat consciously, we feel satisfied and have no desire for food until the next meal, when we naturally begin to feel hungry. Snacking before we are completely hungry gets in the way of our body fully metabolizing the earlier meal. An unmetabolized meal is one of the causes of toxicity in our body.

There are a lot of myths circulating about eating frequent, smaller meals throughout the day. This may be needed for those with blood sugar issues or certain other health conditions. But in general, eating meals at regular times will go a long way towards improving our health and maintaining our focus. It is useful to have even a vague idea of what your meal will be, instead of randomly eating whatever is around. That leads to mindless eating and does not provide the satisfaction that we desire on every level. When it comes to our health, short-term thinking results in short-term health; for long-term health we must think about the long term effects of our habits

5. PAUSE BEFORE GIVING IN TO CRAVINGS

As mentioned earlier, emotional eating tends to be automatic and virtually mindless. Before you even realize what you're doing, you've reached for a tub of ice cream and polished off half of it. But if you can take a moment to pause and reflect when you are hit with a craving, you give yourself the opportunity to make a different decision.

All you have to do is put off eating for five minutes, or if five minutes seems unmanageable, start with one minute. Don't tell yourself you can't give in to the craving; remember, the forbidden is extremely tempting. Just tell yourself to wait. Sip on a cup of tea or a glass of water. Grab an orange. While you're waiting, check in with yourself. How are you feeling? What's going on emotionally? Even if you end up eating, you'll have a better understanding of why you did it. This can help you set yourself up for a different response next time. It may take you a few tries to clue in as to whether or not your hunger is related to your emotions. Anything you eat outside of your meals is worth paying attention to.

Our body is highly intelligent, however we can definitely undermine that intelligence if we stuff our cravings with fatty and sugary snacks. Cravings tend to hit between meals, especially if our meals are missing the nutrients and tastes our body needs. In fact, cravings are indicative of an imbalance in our physiology. In my clinical practice, I have noticed an interesting association between the tastes my clients crave and their psychological implications.

Here's what I have discovered: sweet cravings point to the need for nurturance or love in our lives. Salty or spicy cravings may point to the need of adding some spice or zing to our lives. Cravings for bitter foods may be due to the need to digest the bitter in our lives, perhaps our own bitterness. Cravings for astringent tastes may point to the need to set boundaries, and cravings for pungent foods means we need to experience a kick, or more passion, in our life. Cravings for sour taste may indicate a need to be more flexible or adaptable to life's ups and downs. Don't take this too seriously, but it may help you to think beyond your cravings.

6. AVOID EXTREMES

Extremes tend to present one of the major challenges in our relationship with food. Whether we are dealing with guilt, shame, or other emotions, we very often end up in a state of either overconsumption or utter rigidity in our diets. We continue to swing like a pendulum from one extreme to the other. Here are my thoughts on why this is so: extremes give us a solution, a short-term one and a misguided one, but a solution nonetheless. We know what to do when we are taking an all-or-nothing approach to our food. Either way, we don't need to think, we simply follow the path we've laid out for ourselves.

Thinking and figuring out food-related solutions without a logical, pre-determined system to guide us is challenging to our mind. When we can't figure it out, we give up and do what's easiest. We have all been there, at least I know I have. As I mentioned earlier, we mess up our body's intelligence by ignoring it. The way to restore it is to go deeper than the craving and satisfy it by adding real nutrients to our meals. When our body and mind are balanced, we actually can eat whatever we want, as what we want is the same thing as what our body needs. When we understand and honor our body's innate intelligence, we can reap its benefits.

Doesn't that sound like a self-functioning fool-proof system? It was certainly designed that way. Our body communicates to us and we listen to it. Our eating lines up with what our body needs. We become intuitive, our body responds and remains intelligent, and we become even more intuitive. This is how living and eating is meant to be. Our long term objective is for our whole being to function cohesively. How do we get to that stage? We begin where we are, as we are, with a small tiny step in the direction of following our own intelligence.

If you are curious about how your relationship with food might be affecting your overall health and wellbeing, then I invite you to complete the questionnaire on my website. It will help you think a little more deeply about where you are in your healing journey and perhaps give you a few things to consider as you read the rest of this book. You can find it here: https://www.ayurvedichealingcenter.com/ayurveda/initial-consulation-questionnaire/.

It isn't that we don't know what's right and wrong for us. It is just that we don't do the right thing, even when we know we should.

Our body is always trying to achieve homeostasis; a point of equilibrium in all its functioning. It is always a balancing act. Balance is how we want to think when it comes to food. Not too much and not too little—the middle ground, where growth happens. We want to lean towards the middle ground and have an easy relationship with food. Do you love chocolate? Enjoy it in moderation. You seldom need the whole bar. A couple of squares will do. No food should be taboo if you enjoy it. Avoiding what you love will take you to the other extreme of binging on it. Moderation is key. When you become too strict with food i.e. "I will never ever eat _____," the urge to break that rule will grow just as strong because we have something called an ego, the culprit that keeps us stuck. (Mind you, it can be a blessing if we understand how to use it!) Finding the middle ground is the answer to many of our challenges in life and if we can become comfortable getting to that place, we will grow tremendously and find the inner peace and love that we are ultimately seeking (we'll talk more about that later).

As I mentioned earlier, we can start with one step that we feel we can do. This will take us to the next step, and so forth. All the tools given here are interdependent and not mutually exclusive. Following one technique will help you with another. For example, writing in your food and mood journal, and exploring your beliefs about food, will raise your awareness to the point where you may no longer care to indulge in the extremes, but can find a middle ground.

7. ASSESS YOUR LIFESTYLE

It is rarely the case that our struggles are only with food. We show up as we are in all areas of our life. Our struggles with food have less to do with food and more to do with us, as in, how we are being or showing up in our lives. In other words, our struggles are not isolated, rather they are related to the whole of our life. My clients don't just have digestion issues, they have issues with "digesting" their lives.

Our lifestyle has to do with how we live, how we think, how we relate to others and to Nature, and how we are being in our communities. Our sleeping habits, our emotional habits and our relationship habits are all connected. When we make a change to improve one thing—let's say our sleep habits— we improve our emotional health and our relationships. This is real medicine. How is your sleep? Both the quantity and the quality matter. Sleep deprivation leads to over-indulgence in sugary and fatty foods, not to mention caffeine. What about your shopping habits, particularly your grocery shopping habits? What's in your pantry and fridge? We won't eat healthily if we don't shop healthily. Who cooks in your home? What about relationships? This is another big area that affects our health. *One of my clients had chronic back pain which disappeared once she decided to leave her toxic relationship.* Are you happy with your career? What else is unresolved in your life that may be pulling you down? As you do this self-inquiry, you may notice patterns of behavior repeating in all areas of your life. This may give you a clearer picture of what the real issues are, which may be far bigger than just food.

It is clear that our food struggles are not limited to food. Food struggles are indicative of other bigger struggles in your life that also need resolving. When we begin to heal one area of our life, we heal the whole of our life; it happens naturally and simultaneously. No extra effort is required but allowance is a must. In the meantime, you can find some gentle, healthy ways to soothe yourself other than with food. Feeling exhausted? Take a hot bath or a nap. Set up a bedtime routine. Have a cup of tea. Light some candles. Slow down and just be. Sit with a warm blanket and a cup of tea and enjoy looking out the window. Feeling anxious and worried? Learn to pray. Create an altar in your home to "physicalize" your prayers. Talk to a friend, go for a walk. You get the picture. You can do this, one tiny step at a time!

8. MOVE, MOVE, AND MOVE

I can't stress this enough! Our body represents the sub-stratum of our mind. Moving and breathing is how we circulate the energy of stagnant thoughts and feelings and help them transform. Without involving our body, we can't experience freedom or peace, we can only talk about it. Both breathing and meditating are inner movements that do the trick. Outer movements which engage the physical body, such as walking, running, swimming, yoga, biking, playing sports, and gym activities are all wonderful ways to move.

Everything is energy and frequency is one way to measure it. Our thoughts and emotions are also energy. A sedentary body creates a different thought than a body that is in motion. Give it a try! Difficulty getting out of bed in the morning is a classical symptom of depression. The body has been mostly still during sleep at night, but the situation gets better once the person begins to move. Going for a brisk walk can immediately change your mood.

A body in motion gives motion to your thoughts and feelings, allowing them to transform. One of the principles of energy is that like attracts like. The more we remain stuck in our negative thoughts and emotions, the more of the same we attract into our life. To change our outer environment, we need to change the inner environment i.e. the energy of our body.

We can't feel different from the experience of our body at the cellular and molecular level. It is this environment that we need to change, and we can change it by moving, breathing and meditating. Negative emotions may arise, but they won't hold your interest. They won't stick, as they no longer match the vibration of the inner environment. This is one of the reasons why talk therapy is not sufficient to bring about a lasting change. We can't talk our way through our challenges, we must experience a different way of being and know that there is something else that is available for us to feel. Meditation (a way to build mental stamina) and physical exercise (a way to build physical stamina) are both powerful ways to effect change in the mind.

Put the technology to good use here. Find an app for walking, dancing, meditating or whatever you fancy. I am sure there is an app for it. I frequently use a running app that trains me in interval running. There are group classes of all kinds out there—try them. Find one that you like. Switch things around so your routine holds your interest. Take charge, this is your opportunity!

Every now and then as the need may be, I meet clients at a nearby running track for their follow-up appointment. I check on the progress they've made since the previous week, inquire as to what worked and what didn't, and discover what the obstacles to success for them were, if any, all while we are walking together around the track. Before they know it, they are stretching, doing jumping jacks or shuffles and much more. An hour goes by quickly. They sweat, breathe and move. The end result is that they feel better, which affects their eating and food choices, and that inspires them to do more. For the same reasons, I will also schedule follow-ups in my kitchen. Sometimes, we need a little taste of how we *can* feel, and that gets us inspired to do more. So, even if you hate moving, try it one time and give it your all, and allow yourself a different experience of yourself. You just might like it!

9. ENGAGE IN YOUR LIFE

Developing an interest in all that matters to our health tends to keep that which is not healthy away. Having curiosity about how food can heal or how to cook healthily are some of the ways we can engage in our lives. Being engaged isn't about being busy or distracted, rather it is about immersing yourself in something so much that it fulfills you.

In a world filled with entertainment, excitement and options, we have forgotten—or we devalue—the simple things that we must do. Finding the extraordinary in an ordinary life is the ultimate sophistication, where we can engage in the ordinary day-to-day tasks of cooking our meals, cleaning up after ourselves, and simply sitting and doing our work, instead of constantly looking to distract ourselves. Being endlessly busy does not necessarily get us anywhere.

We don't always have to paint the town red or have a blast with our friends. More often than not, we need to be fulfilled just being with ourselves. There is something that happens when we are totally comfortable in our own skin and can be totally engaged in ourselves. We become creative, we get to know ourselves, we become introspective. This de-stresses our nervous system, gives it an opportunity to digest our life, unwind, and, in turn, it reduces our stress.

The easiest thing to do is to be endlessly distracted with a list of meaningless to-do's that fail to bring fulfillment into our lives. When we are not internally engaged, we seek distractions, and food offers that distraction. Food can provide an instant gratification, a feeling of love and warmth. We can over-focus on food when we don't have much else going on in our lives.

I have found that when our lives are purpose-driven, we are not overly focused on food all the time but eat according to what we need. Again, the solution lies in evaluating your life from a larger context and assessing where the gaps are. Learning to cultivate presence of mind, patience and grace is worth the effort. Doing what is easy makes life harder in the future; doing what's right may be harder in the short term, but it makes life easier in the long run.

Boredom is not necessarily about the lack of a to-do list, it is the inability of the mind to immerse or engage in what we are doing. Interestingly enough, this has become more of a modern-time phenomenon than it ever used to be. We are over-stimulated and entertained to the extent that we have forgotten how to just "be." Seemingly engaged, we are totally disengaged from ourselves.

The nature of the mind is such that it wants to be somewhere other than where it is! It continuously seeks enjoyment and entertainment. But the good news is, our mind can be entertained by anything. We can be totally engrossed in watching a bug, a TV show or cutting our toenails. In other words, the activity does not matter to the mind. It is our ability to engage in whatever it is that we are doing that matters. It is nothing more than a perception that one thing is more exciting than another. As long as the mind is engaged, it is excited, which is why each of us finds that different things are exciting and fun. The point is that the more we engage on an internal level, the more we will move in a healthy direction in all aspects of our life.

There was a lot in this chapter. What point stuck out for you that you would like to explore?

CHAPTER 3

Our Disconnection from Food

As many of my clients turn their health around with food and other lifestyle changes, they desire for their loved ones to do the same. They often share with me the comments that they are met with:

"Oh, I don't believe in this food stuff."

"You mean I had a bad night with my knee pain because I ate all those cupcakes? Are you crazy?"

People continue to believe that a pill is the only answer to their health issues and, as a result, they perpetualize their illnesses through their eating habits. It's bad enough that we don't link illness to our food intake; what's worse is that we believe that only a pill can bring the cure. How did this come to be?

The strong marketing of drugs convinces many of us that no matter what we're suffering from—whether it's heartburn, chronic pain, or the common cold—there is a pill for it. Regardless of all the side effects that the law forces drug companies to disclose in their marketing, what stands out for consumers is the powerful connection between an illness and the drug that promises to make it go away.

We don't really *hear* the side effects when they're named in a TV ad because the drug companies don't want us to hear them. Notice how quickly the side effects are read out to a vulnerable audience desperately seeking relief from their symptoms? Coincidentally, on your next visit to the doctor's office, he/she just happens to have that very same pill, a sample at that, and free to you. As you will read several times throughout the book, our subconscious beliefs are subtle, yet powerful, and by repeatedly watching these ads, we are allowing drug companies to change our subconscious beliefs.

REVERSING YOUR RESULTS

What also stands out for me is that pharmaceutical ads start out with the illness already in place and accepted as a fact of life, as if we were just born with it. There is no talk of *how* the illness came to be, and therefore nothing about what you, the viewer can do to reverse the conditions that led to it. You are deemed powerless as "they" are the only ones with a solution to your problem; hence the blind faith in the pill remains, even when the results are not achieved. The advertisers throw out another hook and a psychological carrot is dangled before you, perhaps someone is dancing happily, or there is a fun scene with friends, a grandchild is swung up onto grandpa's shoulders. Even when no one gets that carrot from the pill, the desire for it is lit.

Modern medicine and pills are the answers to acute illnesses, where the question is about life and death. Modern medicine saves lives every single day. The question is, do we want to be living at the edge of life and death? Is that what we want to deal with in our life? I think not! We want to thrive, be totally alive and do what we came here to do.

In order to have energy, vitality and health, we can't outsource our health to someone else.

Go to the doctor when you need help in managing your disease. But our goals are much higher. When we don't have disease, there is nothing to manage. When we don't have disease, what we do have is energy and time to live our best and most desired life. And those goals are not lofty, they are within your reach. The question is, are you ready for that?

This disconnect between what we eat and the illnesses we develop is alarming and highly concerning. Not only will this keep us sick, but it will keep the next generation sick as well, as our children absorb the information about diet and health that we pass on to them. As if that were not enough, our blind faith in modern medicine leaves us vulnerable: in inviting others to take charge of our health, we rob ourselves of our power to protect it. It is my sincere hope that we will all wake up and think for ourselves when it comes to our health. With that idea in mind, we owe it to ourselves to ask this one question: "How did I get here?"

THE ANSWERS ARE IN YOUR KITCHEN

The answers to chronic illness lie in your kitchen and your lifestyle, and they are therefore in your hands and within your reach. Food has been used from the beginning of time to heal, to prevent disease and to create a vibrant life. This isn't a "New Age" phenomenon: food is our oldest and most effective medicine and it has stood the test of time. It will serve you to pay attention to that and turn the ads off!

Luckily our body is forgiving, to an extent. As soon as we begin to feed it well, it responds. Food works whether you believe it or not. Eat junk and create illness; eat real food and create health! It's just that simple!

Start now!

Inflammation is at the root of most, if not all, illnesses of the body and mind. All processed food causes inflammation, with sugar being the biggest culprit. What is the one food that you can eliminate? Eliminate it for a few days and notice any difference in your pain level, energy level, mood and ability to relax. With each processed food product, you eliminate, you can add a healthy yummy food to your repertoire. You can continue this until you entirely clean your diet. Even if you get rid of only one item per month, you can get rid of 12 disease-causing items from your food in a year and within a year, you can potentially regain your health. Now you can form experiential-based beliefs about food and your health.

As an aside for those who don't believe that food can heal you, please consider this: when you take a pill, it goes through the esophagus and down to the stomach to the small and then the large intestine. Along the way, many mechanical and chemical processes have to take place in order for this pill's journey to deliver the essential chemicals to the targeted area. Well, food follows the same pathway and the natural vitamins and minerals and medicinal properties of the food get transferred to your body via the same mechanism. So, you believe in a pill but not in food? Why is that?

Is there a special mysterious path that the pill follows that we don't know about? All drugs and pills are created for one of two reasons:

1. To duplicate the natural functions of the body that are no longer working and/or
2. To negate our body's natural responses to our lifestyle.

Without adjusting our lifestyle and eating to restore our body's natural intelligence, we must depend on the pill forever and suffer the side effects, not to mention the fact that we miss out on a huge opportunity to learn and take charge of our own health. The fact is that the innate intelligence of our body remains. We can access it. It is like the sun that is always there, even on cloudy days. And we can tap into that natural intelligence. It is far easier and natural to do that than to "chemicalize" our body and suffer in the long run. Our healing isn't separate from our eating and living; when we change how we eat and how we live, we are creating an inner environment of healing.

SMOOTHIES

It seems that if we are not totally disconnected from food, we are obsessed with it and I need to say a few words about smoothies, our modern-day food invention. We find all the power foods, combine them together and literally dump them into our bodies via our morning smoothie. When we bypass many of the important functions, such as chewing, that turn on our digestion, we undermine our body's intelligence and we don't achieve the results that we may have anticipated. As much as we may want to, we can't outsmart Nature.

Stacie came to me suffering from bloating that lasted throughout the day but was especially bad after breakfast. I discovered that she was making smoothies out of what she believed to be all good stuff, and she was making enough to last for three or four days as a way to save time. Right off the bat, I knew that this was causing her bloating: too many ingredients were being mixed together at once, and the food wasn't fresh after the first serving. It was fermenting, making it unsuitable for consumption. Although Stacie was trying to eat healthily and save time, her effort did not work. As soon as she stopped the smoothies and replaced them with a warm, cooked breakfast, the bloating went away.

We are swimming in information about what we should be eating every day to remain healthy, and

27

there is a lot of good food available to us. Getting all of what we need sometimes feels like a full-time job. None of us can keep up with that. So, it seems easy to dump all the goodness we can find into one single drink and stop worrying about it. Can't figure out a way to incorporate superfoods into your diet? Eating on the run all the time? No worries, just toss all the goodies you can find into your smoothie!

Here's the catch: the most organic and nutrient-dense ingredients don't operate the way we might expect. Mixing many different textures and tastes, and combining foods that should not be combined, undermines the intelligence of the body and we pay the price in the long run.

But there's something else wrong with this picture!

When we drink our meals, we don't chew them. Chewing is one of the most important triggers for turning on our digestive juices. Chewing allows you to experience eating, and chewing longer changes the taste of food to sweetness. What's more, when we add too many ingredients into our smoothie—and especially ones that don't combine well—we are launching an assault on our digestive system.

TREAT YOUR BODY GENTLY

Morning is not a good time to drink your food. Your body is still in "fasting mode" after the previous night's dinner and it has been busy digesting, cleansing and eliminating (at the cellular level) while we were sleeping. When you awaken in the morning, your body needs to be treated gently. It needs something warm and gentle, such as oatmeal, a cooked apple, fresh toast with nut butters, eggs, hot tea, etc. We can have smoothies later on in the day if we choose, but keep the following in mind so they deliver the goodness that you are after:

1. Fruits and vegetables should not be combined in a smoothie as your body digests fruit much faster than vegetables. But food stays in the stomach until the last ingredient is digested and processed, so fruit sugar from a smoothie will start fermenting the vegetables before they are fully digested. This creates bloating, gas and toxicity in the gut.

2. Most greens are bitter and astringent in taste and they are both catabolic (which means they promote a process which breaks down tissues) and cooling. To introduce them in the morning when your body needs gentle nourishment affects your ability to metabolize food throughout the rest of the day.

3. Drinking too much raw (uncooked) green vegetables aggravates the Air and Space element, or Vata, and we'll talk about these issues later in the book. Moreover, ingesting raw and cold food like these reduces the efficiency of our digestion.

4. Long-term dependence on smoothies generally leads to nutritional depletion, even if you may notice a power surge in the short term after you drink one; many of my clients have ended up feeling sick despite quaffing a power smoothie daily.

5. Adding nut butters and extra fats to smoothies makes them difficult to digest and ultimately will create toxins in your body, instead of the nourishment that you had intended.

If you enjoy smoothies and want to include them in your diet, incorporating some of the tips below will help you obtain the benefit you seek from them.

1. Think of the smoothie as a snack and not a substitute for a meal. So, mid-afternoon is a good time to drink one, if you are hungry.

2. Make either a green smoothie or a fruit smoothie. Avoid combining the two.

3. Making a smoothie with just two or three different fruits is okay such as berries and mango, or berries and pineapple.

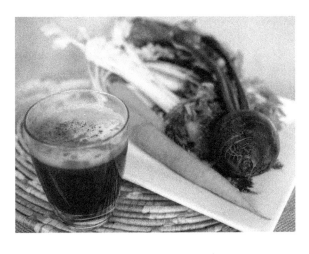

4. Drink your smoothie at room temperature.

5. Add water instead of coconut or almond milk

6. Far better than a green smoothie is to eat your greens cooked, rather than raw. Sauté them lightly in ghee (clarified butter) with the spice mix. (See recipe in Chapter 16). This will give you all the benefits without any of the drawbacks.

7. Try celery, carrot and beet juice as a tonic and energy boost. (4-6 stalks of celery, 2-3 carrots, ½ a beet)

OUR DISCONNECTION FROM FOOD SOURCE

Where does our food come from? How does it end up in our local grocery store? How is it produced? Who produces it?

Right at the corner of my subdivision, there is a beautiful mulberry tree. It is as healthy as can be as it gets full sunlight and it has a lot of space to grow. The tree is full of berries throughout the summer months. I often stop by the tree on my walks and grab a few handfuls of berries to enjoy. One day, a man driving by stuck his head out his car window and asked, "Can you eat those?" I answered, "I hope so, because I am eating them!" Then he said, "My wife won't go near them as she does not trust food right off of the trees."

So, this is where we are when it comes to knowing the source of our food! We happily buy food from grocery stores without question, but won't trust it right off of the tree, its source. The one thing we can do is trust food we have picked right from its source. It is what's in the store that needs our attention and discernment. The path from the tree to the grocery store is what we must question and understand. We know crops are treated with pesticides. We just don't know much about their impact on our health. Much of that information is coming out now. The further the food grows from our home, the more it's treated with chemicals to sustain its "freshness." Some of it may be necessary, and some is clearly overdone. The best thing to do is buy organic and locally grown food wherever possible.

THE PROTEIN CONUNDRUM

Another big concern surrounds meat products and how they are produced. If nothing else would make us question our dietary habits, then the link between meat consumption and disease should wake us up. The National Cancer Institute[2] has linked red meat consumption to cancer, heart disease, respiratory disease, stroke, diabetes, infections, kidney disease, and liver disease. The link to disease is not just because of the chemicals applied while the animals are still alive and then again after they are killed, it is also as a result of the cruelty imposed on these animals

Animal cruelty in the production of meat is not an unknown subject. We conveniently ignore it, as, what can we do about it, anyway? Giving up foods that we have come to love is something we are not willing to do. And, in particular, if this has been a way of living for you, changing it may not feel possible. Nonetheless, it is worth knowing how the meat that we consume is produced and what path it has taken on its way to our dinner plate.

Animals are force-fed, treated heavily with chemicals, confined, and killed in the most inhumane ways possible, all so we can have our protein. We justify it because we feel we need what we need. A few things are noteworthy here. Our lives are far more important than the lives of these animals, yet we consume them in the hopes of completing our nourishment. How is that possible? On the surface, this may seem only a moral issue. It is far more than that, as the moral issue affects our spirituality and in turn our healing. Yes, spirituality and healing are not separate things, they are one and the same. When I talk about health, I am talking about more than our physical health. Health here is all-encompassing, and includes our spiritual health. By switching to organic meat, we may improve its quality, but the moral dilemma still remains, which affects our spirituality, our healing, and our Karma. And we can rationalize it in any way possible to justify our actions. Whether we can justify it or not does not have anything at all to do with the effect it has on our health.

We are all familiar with the laws of Karma, which suggest you "Do onto others as you want done to you," and we remember that "What goes around, comes around." When we treat life unkindly, we are treating ourselves unkindly, it is that simple. We can't sustain life by taking life; we can't experience kindness when all we have imparted is cruelty. Denial, or pretending this isn't so, does not make a difference to the law of Karma. It is a simple science of action and reaction or cause and effect. What we do to Nature, we do to ourselves, as we are not separate from it. This is how it works, whether we like it or not.

With every bite of meat, we also ingest pain and suffering, as that is the energy that is in the meat. Along with protein, the pain and suffering becomes our pain and suffering. We are part of the whole of Creation. The abuse of animals leads to the abuse of our kindness, our heart and our Consciousness. This creates a huge disconnect from the source of our food and a total disconnect from our own Source. We are so far removed from the source of our food that we pretend that it does not matter how it got to our table. We pretend that the abuse of animals is irrelevant just because we did not directly cause it.

We may not see animals' pain, but we can surely feel it. If you truly desire to find out what's going on with your "food," a trip to the slaughterhouse will do the trick. In spite of technological advancements, there is endless suffering in the world and an epidemic of disease. This is not a coincidence. Everything affects everything else. Life for life; when we take life, we sow the seed of our own demise. Because we are all connected and made of the same stuff, we are part of the collective Karma.

Please understand that Karma is not a judgement or punishment from the Creator. It is simply an energy that is created through our actions. We create Karma (good and bad) every moment in our lives by our thoughts, by what we do and what we say. What's needed is for us to take responsibility for the Karma we create. This can be a great motivator to mindful living on all levels. Good Karma creates positive energy and bad Karma creates negative or dark energy. Both the energies are part and parcel of our being.

The objective is to transmute the dark energy into love. Another way of understanding is to accept our own darkness and in the accepting, we expand more into who we are: Love! Darkness is as much a part of love and light, it is in accepting and owning our darkness, that we move to light. So, we don't use Karma to control others, rather to point out the result of our actions, as every action creates a reaction and this process is explained by Karma. Anything more than what is explained here is beyond the scope of this book and, frankly, beyond my own understanding.

And is the cost of meat production worth its benefits? Not to mention the psychological effects on those who are at the front line of producing it. So, these are some of the issues to consider if we want to consume meat. We can't expect healing from acts of violence to life—all of life. This may not be convenient. Truth seldom is!

This is what connecting to our food source looks like. It requires Consciousness and our willingness to look beyond what's on our dinner plate. Introspection of one's life and life choices has never hurt anyone. Taking a life may not kill us immediately but it sure kills something like our humanity, empathy, love and kindness. It sure is a death of "honoring all life" and harmonizing with the whole of Creation.

FEEL DEEPLY, THINK DEEPLY, LOVE DEEPLY

This deep connection with what surrounds us, with Nature and all life is a way of deeper connection with ourselves. We can't continue to live a superficial life and expect deep transformation. Our life journey is to feel deeply, think deeply and love deeply because we can afford to. We can always afford to care more and love more.

To give up foods that we have come to love is never easy. As mentioned earlier, instead of taking an "all-or-nothing" approach, the point is to become more conscious and understand that food is the source of our energy and the energy of our food affects our own energy. In that way of thinking, you are already starting to think beyond what's on your dinner plate. This opens up a lot more possibilities and choices for you than you may have originally thought. We have free will, we can do what we choose. But it would be wise to choose with an expanded awareness.

I questioned whether to include this chapter in this book as I want to offer you the most unbiased thought process that I can. Will it disturb those of us who do eat meat? Is there something really wrong with eating meat? After all, we are all in this circle of life and death. Perhaps the killing of animals for meat consumption is a way to control the animal population and it is what Nature wants? Well, I believe that Nature has built in ways to control both the animal and the human population. Who are we to decide if there are too many animals on this planet? Frankly, there is an overpopulation of us humans in the world, are we going to take that into our own hands, too? Secondly, I believe that which gave life, *all* life, has the lone right to take it. Life and death are better left in the hands of the Creator. And that, my friends, is neither you nor me. Whether you eat meat on not, I firmly believe that we won't get far by torturing and killing animals. Our health and healing is directly related to it.

The protein worry isn't real. Being a vegetarian all my life, I have never worried about having enough protein, or lacking energy and strength. I participated in sports and even today remain quite physically active. I share this with you to break the myth that meat is the only source of protein. Massive protein intake from animal products is not necessary for good health and, in fact, there is growing evidence to indicate it can actually be quite harmful to us.

The belief that we need large amounts of meat protein is imparted to us from a very young age by our culture and it is reinforced with near-constant exposure to officially-sanctioned national food guides and food pyramids. We must pay attention to the source of these guidelines and question whether they are really are in the best interest of our health. Animal products such as fish, dairy, eggs and meat are marketed as the only complete source of protein and are based on a "one-size-fits-all" approach to nutrition. They give no consideration to issues that are key to a holistic view of health, such as an individual's age, gender, unique constitution, state of balance, state of mind, or distinct level of spiritual awareness.

So many of the health issues that I encounter in my practice are directly related to meat consumption. When my clients move to a more plant-based diet, they get healthier. Some of the results they experience include weight loss, higher energy, mental clarity, better sleep, normalized blood pressure, decreased pain and an overall sense of well-being. In addition, many of my female clients experience a reduction in hot flashes and normalized menstrual cycles.

While there are many illnesses that are linked to meat consumption, I have yet to find an illness that comes from being vegetarian. It is, however, important to note that the vegetarian diet may create some deficiencies including vitamin B12. Consider evaluating your whole diet and adding supplements where needed.

Consider the following if you want to lean towards a more plant-based diet.

1. Have a day without meat and see how you feel.
2. Eat meat at lunch time only. Notice the effect on your sleep.
3. Reduce meat portion size and combine it with plenty of leafy greens.
4. Cook meat with digestive spices. (See the recipe for this in Chapter 16)

Skip meat for two days with a goal of eventually eating it perhaps couple of times a week, or once in a while. Trust your experiences and give your body some time to adjust.

There are many vegetarian sources of protein. While this is not a complete list, here are a few I use most routinely in my diet:

- All lentils and beans, chick peas, black eyed peas
- Grains such as quinoa and amaranth
- Green peas, artichokes, edamame, spinach, broccoli, asparagus, green beans, all leafy greens
- Nuts and seeds such as almonds, walnuts, pumpkin seeds, hemp hearts, chia seeds
- Nut butters including tahini
- Nutritional yeast, spirulina powder

Our culture of extremes and indulgences makes us perfect targets for manipulation, make-believe, and marketing, and if we want a balanced and complete view of what our nutritional needs truly are, we need to lean heavily on our common sense, wisdom and intelligence. We need to replace our old nutritional paradigm with one that is holistically devoted to our health. Paying attention to the changing seasons, your body's changing needs, and the wisdom of Nature will promote long-term health and vitality.

The changing seasons provide natural dietary guidance, if we are willing to pay attention. The wisdom and truth of Mother Nature points us to a high-protein, high-fat diet in winter, a very low-fat diet in the spring, a high-carbohydrate diet in summer that is heavy on veggies, fruits and grains, and back to a little heavier diet as fall begins. Spring is the logical time to restrict calories as it forces the body to reset its ability to use fat as a primary source of fuel. In essence, a low-fat diet in spring forces our body to burn its own fat, which is the goal of a ketogenic diet, our latest diet fad. Any diet can be a medicinal diet in the short term, however when the desired results are achieved, we must get off that diet.

WHAT ABOUT DAIRY?

The treatment of animals isn't any better when it comes to milk and dairy production. Treated like milk-producing machines, cows are plugged in to milking machines, they are force-fed and they are heavily drugged with chemicals. The "motherly" qualities that milk was revered for are no longer available in the way milk is produced today.

In India, cows are sacred and often a common household animal; they are part of the family. As a result, milk is revered and it's synonymous with mother, nurturance and love. We always had a cow while we were growing up. Our cow was loved and cared for. She had a big room in a barn set in the shade and a nice breeze blew through to keep her comfortable. She had a big open space for walking in the evenings and she had warm blankets at night. She was bathed, fed and milked, and she was taken care of well. In return, her milk nurtured the whole family and we enjoyed fresh butter every morning.

Whenever our cow heard my dad come home, she would not settle until he came to see her. He would pet her and chat with her. She was a happy cow, and she would stand quietly and peacefully while being milked. I grew up drinking hot, boiled milk at bed time. Milk was rarely consumed cold, unless it was a really hot day. Then we would put water into the raw milk and add ice and sugar to make a cooling drink. I still enjoy the nutritive qualities of milk I purchase from a local dairy farm.

We do what we can. There is no judgement on whether you eat meat or not, drink milk or not. If you wish to consume milk, you may want to follow a few guidelines below to make it digestible. Most allergies to milk stem from its wrongful consumption.

- Buy only organic or raw milk if possible. Get it from a reputable source that you know cares for their cows with kindness.
- Never drink milk cold but rather dilute it with water (50/50), add a few slices of fresh ginger root, and bring it all to a boil first. Once you can tolerate it, then you may not have to dilute it so much.
- Don't drink milk with salty food as it will curdle, and upset your stomach.
- Don't combine milk with yogurt, meat, cheese or eggs.
- Don't drink milk at mealtime. It is a great bedtime treat, as it is natural sleep aid and a laxative.

How we live and how we eat is not separate from how we heal. I encourage all of my clients to keep an open mind and see if you can connect a little more with the foods you consume to determine how they affect your health and well-being. All you need to do is pay attention, it does not require more time. Attention takes as much time as inattention and it may give you a sense of deeper connection and a sense of responsibility for your part in it. We make the world what it is! Each one of us matters. Avoid the all-or-nothing approach as it tends to be temporary. Gain a deeper understanding instead. Do what you can today and this can change the direction of your health.

Think about a health issue that you may be having and see if it has a connection to what you are eating by eliminating or reducing "that" food.

CHAPTER 4

Overconsumption and Addiction

We are a culture of overconsumption. If a little is good, more must be better. Big boys, big meals, free refills, extra-large fries, all-we-can-eat buffets, Costco and all-inclusive vacations are all part of our lifestyle. We are getting sicker as a nation in more ways than one. Do we have too much?

Having too much can affect us in one of two ways. It can create an abundance mindset which means we feel secure and grateful with everything we have and happily share it with others. This keeps the flow going, making us all feel abundant. Or it can make us feel insecure and fearful of losing it. We begin to hoard like pigs in mud, as if we have never seen an item before and, who knows, we may never get it again! This creates a "hungry ghost" as, regardless of how much we have, we feel we don't have enough, and we therefore continue to overconsume. It's for each one of us to figure out our own mindset and move in the direction of feeling abundant and secure.

It takes more than skill to navigate the culture of overconsumption and stay true to our own goals and aspirations. What's needed is a complete internal rewiring, and a deep mindfulness.

I have had my own challenges with overconsumption. Cooking small portions was a big challenge for me as I had always seen food in large quantities due to the large family into which I was born. Even in college days, in spite of both lack of time and funds, when I did cook I would prepare large portions, much more than I needed, and I would share the excess with my landlady. She would enjoy what I had cooked and would say that if I ate this way all the time, I would be very healthy! She had seen me eating on-the-run or forgetting to eat altogether, at which point she would bring a cheese and tomato sandwich up to my room.

I didn't know this was a problem until I was a mom.

I continued to cook large portions but then I would get stressed about having to finish what I had cooked. My sister suggested I freeze the leftovers, which I did, only to realize that some dishes are just not meant to be frozen.

I overcooked because I simply bought too much, which led to the stress of managing, cooking and eating the food. And the reason I bought too much is because I shopped at a very large produce market that not only had a large selection of produce but a large quantity of everything. Being a vegetarian and a food lover, this widened my eyes way bigger than my stomach and I would excitedly and happily buy everything. Although I mostly bought vegetables and fruits, I ended up eating more than I needed simply because I had bought more. Eventually I got a handle on over-buying. I stopped going to the BIG store and learned to buy fresh food every few days instead of stockpiling it as if it were going out of style. Now, I often simply refrain from going to the grocery store until I finish what I have on hand, which forces me to become creative in my kitchen.

Over-consuming food, material things, entertainment or anything else, points to two important issues. First, it means we are making up for an inner lack of something. Our subconscious plays a powerful role in compensating for this lack, and doesn't judge how we are doing that. But as we discussed in Chapter 2, food can't make up for what's missing in our lives. The second thing overconsumption indicates is that we feel somehow insecure about having "enough," even though we may have an abundance of everything in our life. This scarcity mindset makes us greedy and we hoard. The more we have, the more we want. When we have too much, fear of losing it can set in. What if we won't have all this, all the time? Overconsumption of anything can't satisfy our needs, however; it can only be corrected by connecting to our Source.

THE DESIRE FOR "MORE"

To some extent we have all bought into the belief that more is better. There is a certain lure to the bigger home, the bigger car, the bigger refrigerator or an extra freezer, the big screen TV, and the computer or mobile phone with bigger capacity. And still the desire for "more" remains. Perhaps there is a perception that having more confers a higher status and a better quality of life. Or we are trying to overcompensate for not having had enough at some point in our lives. The accumulation of material things, including food, may give us a higher status, but a healthier and happier life is a balanced life. A better life is a healthier life.

Food is everywhere we turn and it has become normal for people to overindulge at social gatherings, and snack non-stop. It is important to point out that we can overconsume healthy food as well, at which point it can become "too much of a good thing." Overconsumption of processed food is a much bigger cause of concern as it creates a deficiency in our body that we then must seek to balance. The average grocery store sells more processed food than fresh, "real" food, which obviously encourages increased consumption of processed food. The more processed food we purchase, the more retailers make available and, as more becomes available, the more we purchase. I contend that the overconsumption of processed food products leads to disease. Prevention is the ultimate cure and that is what we are after when we use food as medicine.

We can thank the marketing world, as well, again, for luring us into overconsumption. The slogan, "the more you buy, the more you save" is true only if you buy more because you NEED it, and because it is going to move you in the direction that you have set for your life and your health. This affects us psychologically. We don't even think to pick just one apple when there are hundreds in a bin. By prepacking quantities of a fruit or vegetable, the stores are suggesting that we buy that amount and, unless we are paying attention, we just follow along, only to realize that we have bought too much when we get home. We can learn from this experience. We can pack our own quantity in a separate bag and buy what we need rather than buying what we are *told* to buy.

More food just does not just take up more space in our refrigerators, it takes up space in our body as well.

DON'T SAVE MONEY. SAVE YOUR HEALTH. BUY LESS!

I hosted a Sufi Saint in my yoga studio a few years ago. His mission was to travel to as many places as he could to spread his love and blessings. Many people showed up to get his blessings. Two stories about his visit come to mind: The Sufi Saint's disciple asked me for water and asked that I only fill the glass half way. He kneeled down in my kitchen next to the sink and with both hands drank the water as if it were the nectar of life. He drank the entire amount. He asked for only what he needed and did not waste a drop.

The Sufi Saint's comments on worry and fear also stuck with me. He pointed to the birds outside and said, "do they have a fridge? They eat when they are hungry and always find their next meal. We have extra freezers in our basements and garages and yet we are worried about our next meal." I find a lot of truth in his words. In Michigan, it is normal to have a couple of snow storms in the winter months. I am always perplexed when I see the long lines at the grocery store a day before the storm. You would think it were Christmas! Everyone is eager to stock up and be ready for the snowstorm. Aren't our kitchens stocked up enough for one day? The storm lasts a day at most. ONE DAY! And the grocery stores are packed!

Instead of rejoicing in the abundance that has been bestowed upon us, we hoard. So, regardless of how much we have, there is a scarcity programming running through our minds and that's what needs to be rewired. We are on this merry-go-round of overconsumption while moving further and further away from real health, happiness and joy! We must get off, and get off quick!

OVERCONSUMPTION AND WEIGHT LOSS

Nearly all of us are trying to lose weight, which means the weight-loss industry is now a multi-billion dollar industry. This is a crucial issue. Weight gain is not just weight gain, it is heart failure, tissue and organ degeneration, depression and anxiety, and missed opportunities. Food can create either disease or health. It is up to us to decide what we want it to do and choose accordingly. Weight gain requires no effort, only mindlessness and lack of responsibility for one's own health; weight loss, on the other hand requires persistent effort, and every ounce of our awareness.

The best way to lose weight is to not put it on in the first place.

OVERCONSUMPTION AND FOOD ADDICTIONS

Overconsumption can easily lead to food addictions, especially if you are consuming sugars or foods that turn into sugars. Refined sugar, processed foods and simple carbohydrates are addictive. Addiction is a norm for us humans. We are all addicted to comforts, conveniences, happiness and life working according to our whims. What happens if we lose the internet for a day, or lose our phone? If we love something, we want more of it all the time. All the ways we discussed in Chapter 2 about overcoming emotional hunger apply to addictions as well. What works is different for everyone. The quickest path to overcome any addictions is to transcend them through meditation. We connect with our Higher Self which is complete and wholesome. When we solidify our connection with that part of ourselves, food becomes a medicine that prevents disease and keeps us vibrant and healthy. This is how we internally rewire.

It is difficult to go against the grain of society. What would it be like if our individual efforts to stay healthy were not undermined by money-minded corporations? We must be a step ahead and keep our wits about us. Food is our ultimate health insurance. More is not better. Here are a few things worth considering.

1. **A heightened awareness is required to tune into our habits and behaviours and especially our needs.** We must develop a habit of making new habits. The same applies to eating habits. Which ones are working and which ones need to be ditched? Much like the paint color in our homes or our wardrobe, habits need a review and an update from time to time. Writing down what we are eating is a great way to know how much we are actually eating, which can give us awareness on what needs changing.

2. **Real food is the answer to food addictions.**
   Much of food addiction relates to junk—processed food products. The middle aisles in most grocery stores are filled with these products. That is your disease in the making. Avoid them.

3. **Buy most of your food from the produce section.**
   Some stores have a natural section where they keep all of their organic food and food products. Remember, the goal of the stores is to improve their bottom line, not your health. Sometimes, they will intentionally place healthy items in the middle aisles to lure you into buying the other food products that are there. Just being aware of that is helpful.

4. **Pick a smaller cart or, better yet, use a shopping basket.**
   You can also take your own reusable bag with you. By doing that you have already set the ceiling on how much you will buy.

5. **At meal times, take only what your two hands can hold.**
   I have found that our physical hunger is satisfied with little food, the extra is to feed out emotional hunger. I heard "The Banquet is in the first bite" often during my studies, and I remind myself and my clients of this often. It really reminds us to increase our presence and therefore our enjoyment of our food. Taking time to sit down and enjoy a meal without distractions will not only give us more satisfaction but also the time needed for our digestion to work well (we'll talk more about that later!). Bringing awareness to the taste, texture, aroma and color of your food, and being in gratitude for the working hands that made it possible for it to be on your table, will make eating a wholesome experience and will satisfy you more than in just the physical sense. You can always take more if you still desire it.

6. **Use a smaller plate and bowl for your meals.**
   Skipping meals leads to eating more as our body needs the calories to function. When we skip a meal with the hopes of losing weight, we more than make up for it at the next meal. It is better to eat a small meal than to skip it altogether.

7. **Find other ways to soothe yourself.**
   Make self-care your default pattern in any challenge because that is all you can do sometimes. Giving yourself an oil massage, meditating, praying, eating and sleeping on time, reading a book, soaking your feet or soaking in the tub, and going for a walk in Nature are some of the ways to take care of yourself and add sweetness and love into your life.

8. **Lack of movement or exercise leads to overeating.**
   Lack of movement leads to inertia and then we look to food for stimulation. That's when we end up reaching for high-fat and high-sugar foods for a quick energy boost. When our lifestyle is sedentary, we are not likely to chomp on a carrot when hungry. We tend to want heavy foods. But when we are active and have more energy, we don't need the quick energy from food, rather we choose nourishing meals and we tend to eat less. In other words, we choose the foods that match our energy: when we feel heavy and lethargic, we tend to want heavy foods; when we feel energetic, we gravitate towards foods with higher energy, or prana (life force).

9. **Eat to live or live to eat?**

   This is worth pondering. Is food taking center stage in our lives or are we taking center stage with food as an ally that is supporting our life's purpose? What rings true for you? A lack of other interests or passions can make us obsess about food. Pay attention to that. Food is important but it is a means to an end. Food is the fuel that we need to propel forward towards our aspirations and desires. If you find yourself constantly thinking about food, notice if you have other things in your life to hold your interest. Refer to Chapter 2 on the tools to overcome emotional hunger.

It is what we do consistently that matters. Occasional overconsumption is not a problem if we eat in a balanced way most of the time. And, in fact, overconsumption isn't just about food. It could be Netflix, shopping, or something else. Only you can know why you do this—give it some thought. Just simple ways of introspection can give us great insights about our inner world. Life is not about perfection; it is a practice. If you'd like to reflect a little more deeply on your health and your behaviour, it might be helpful to complete the health questionnaire situated on my website: https://www.ayurvedichealingcenter.com/ayurveda/initial-consulation-questionnaire/.

Do you tend towards overdoing things?

Is there a lack in your life of something else?

CHAPTER 5

Lack of Personal Responsibility

Over the course of my career, I have had the privilege of speaking to many groups and organizations and at many events. One event I participated in was for cancer patients and survivors.

This event included a segment where survivors went up on stage and shared their stories of surviving cancer. One survivor shared that she ate her carrots at lunch or dinner, at which point everyone cheered and applauded, and she took a bow. Something about this disturbed me. What seemed like encouragement felt like condescension. It felt to me as though not caring about oneself was the accepted norm and caring about oneself i.e. through eating right was out of the norm and warranted applause. It was like saying, "Oh, isn't it nice that YOU take care of yourself, aren't you special!" Our expectations of others are so low that when someone exceeds our expectations they merit applause. This in a very subtle way sets the societal norm. Our society and the medical world expect that we are too dumb to take care of ourselves.

You eat a carrot and the world applauds! What happens if they don't applaud, do you stop eating your carrot?

At some point in our lives, we must take responsibility for our own health and the rewards are personal and internal. Your health isn't anyone's concern. It must be yours. Taking charge of our health ignites our spirit and lights the path before us, and this is what we give up when we leave our health in someone else's hands.

This event, by the way, was sponsored by a hospital. Coincidentally, at the same event, the breakfast that was served included sugar-glazed cinnamon buns, muffins, donuts and cold cantaloupe or melon for good measure, just to "balance" and "health" things out a little. In serving *that* food to their patients, the hospital made a loud and clear statement: "Food has nothing to do with your illness or your healing." This level of disconnect came right from the custodians and gatekeepers of our health! We are willing to undergo extensive treatments but we are not willing to eat right. We are willing to subject our bodies to drugs and their side effects yet we don't think that what we eat has any bearing on our health at all. This is how disconnected we are. We can't be anything but personally responsible for our health!

We can't outsource our thinking to others. "Tell me what to do exactly and I will follow." "Give me the quick fix so I don't have to deal with life." What seems easy in the beginning makes life harder in the end. What feels harder in the beginning can make our life easier. Don't follow! Lead, instead, by example! Taking responsibility means educating yourself; learning how to live and eat; speaking up when all your doctor does is hand you a script for drugs; demanding more from yourself and your life and living up to your potential. This is what is needed in these times. Sooner or later we must assume responsibility and take charge of our own health. Anything less than that will leave us wide open and a target for money makers where our illness becomes their opportunity; our ignorance provides a way in for them to sell us the path they have already laid out for us, the path of drugs, specialists, and testing when it may not be what we needed to begin with.

Over 15 years ago, I injured my shoulder while practicing a hand stand with my friend, another Yoga teacher. I didn't realize at that time that I had injured it and there wasn't much pain. But my shoulder did not work the same and slowly I lost the full range of movement, which started to distort my alignment. Not knowing what this was, I compensated by overdoing things with my other arm and made it all worse to the point where it hurt just to touch the shoulder. This disrupted my sleep and made other functions of my life like driving and putting a seat belt on very difficult. Finally, I went to a doctor and he told me that there was calcification in the shoulder joint and then he just very casually scheduled a surgery. He said that surgery would be no big deal and they would remove the calcification.

Surgery had never even occurred to me until he scheduled it for me. I liked this doctor and he meant well. This happened so quickly that I was left dumbfounded and confused. I had gone in to find out what was wrong with my shoulder and walked away with a prescription for surgery, all in the matter of 5-10 minutes. I remember thinking that perhaps this is all normal, everyone has surgeries and now it is my turn. I hardly go to the doctor and I didn't tune into my confusion and this cloud that was hanging over my head.

Luckily, I ran into someone who had had a similar surgery more than a year earlier and she was still not healed. She said that what I had was called frozen shoulder. That is the first time I had heard that term. Right then, I sensed that surgery was not my only option. I took matters into my own hand. I needed to know exactly what was wrong with the shoulder, i.e. was something torn? Frozen shoulder could mean a number of things. After ruling all that out with an MRI, I knew what I had to do. With some physical therapy and mostly my own yoga therapy and diet to reduce inflammation, I started to heal my shoulder. Within a year, I was 90% healed and shortly afterwards regained my full range of movement.

Like you, I also thought doctors knew best. I can share many stories with you about healing myself and my son without doctors and now know, in no uncertain terms, that doctors don't know the best option for you, as they only present one option. It is up to us to choose what's best for us.

Healing is not a glamorous or a romantic journey; in fact it can shake you to your core. But it is empowering. And the results are nothing short of miraculous. The well-meaning doctor took my power away by making me believe surgery was the only option. He had an opportunity to educate me, give me options, and inform me of the aftermath of the surgery, and I would have walked away equipped with information on which to base my decision. Instead, he decided for me and used my pain as an opportunity to sell only what he had to offer. He left me confused and disempowered. This is a normal everyday occurrence in the medical world. So, before you rush to a quick fix and hand your health over to someone else, think long and hard. Ask around, look around and get the answers you need.

Feeling confused is a sign to pause and wait until the confusion lifts. You will know when something is right for you. You need to trust that. One of the skills I teach my clients is to trust in their own wisdom. We all know our truth; we just need to trust it and rely on it. Taking the easy way out is actually much harder than doing what's right for you. I had to endure a lot of pain during my recovery but I was okay with it because that is what I chose to do. When we take charge of our own health, something sparks in us; our internal fire and our inner knowing. We come alive and become a force to be reckoned with. Don't let anyone tell you otherwise. After it is all said and done, it is ultimately your life, your health and your responsibility. Anything less than that will leave you open to be victimized.

THE FRESH, HOT, COOKIE TRAP

During the writing of this book, I went out for dinner with my good friend, Sherry, and we talked about the subject of my book. She shared with me something that I thought was very timely and needed to be in the book. It turned out to be the inspiration behind this chapter. Here is what she shared. *In the college town of Ann Arbor, MI, these "insomnia cookies" are all the talk. As the name would suggest, they are targeted to the insomniacs and are delivered "fresh and hot" to college kids in the middle of the night, like at 3:00 a.m.* I checked the company's website before writing this. The menu offers nothing but varieties of cookies like Sugar Rush, Triple Chocolate, Cookie Cake. Etc., and the packaging is quite enticing and attractive. On the surface, this is no big deal; you can get cookies from anywhere. But here is why this is a big deal:

Insomnia or the inability to sleep is an illness that needs treating as it results in other illnesses such as chronic fatigue or adrenal fatigue, mental disorders, depression and anxiety, to name a few. Proper sleep is essential to the healthy functioning of all of the other biorhthyms of our body, and lack of proper sleep makes everything worse. All college kids stay up during the night and do dumb things, but now they can do dumber things and get themselves even sicker just at the touch of a button. There is an opportunity to teach these kids about healthy habits, alternative options and the long term effects of their actions, but instead someone takes this opportunity to make money off of these young people and lead them to a sicker lifestyle. By selling cookies to these kids, they are promoting insomnia and future illness. Sugar is a highly addictive substance which now the kids can get by staying awake. This is why it is of utmost importance that we wake up to our own responsibility in creating the health and the life we desire. And lastly, we must beware of the lure of "hot and fresh." Crap served "hot and fresh" remains crap!

My adult clients who struggle with food addictions and poor eating habits typically ate and lived like that when they were young. Some 30 years later, their way of living in their younger years has resulted in multiple health issues that they can no longer ignore. They struggle with their health and can't seem to do what's healthy, even when they know what to do. The sugar addiction of our youth can leave traces of memory that can get activated in your adult life. These formerly "insomniac kids" can end up as adults who will struggle to stay healthy, and this will mean missed opportunities for them to grow and to live their dreams. What seems like a "norm" can start us on a path of struggle for the rest of our lives. This is no joke and can't be taken lightly.

Loving cookies at 20 can turn into hating your life at 50! Wake up!

Don't let your lack of responsibility be someone else's opportunity. Don't wait to be rescued or saved, as that is your job. Don't look to the outside to decide what the right thing is for you. Don't follow the societal norms when it comes to your health. Don't go with the flow. Don't try to fit into the mainstream, create your own stream. Our reference and guidance must come from within. We are all at a different stage in our life and we all have different lessons to learn. Every life and every situation and every challenge is unique. Fitting in is way over-rated. Fitting in with like-minded people is great, but in order for that to happen; you must know your own mind. Do you agree with whoever you are trying to fit in with? If not, find another group that aligns with you.

Comparing, Conforming and Complaining are the 3 C's to avoid.

Measuring yourself against a world norm is misleading and is not the way to determine what you should do.

A young client thought he should not be too hard on himself for drinking alcohol three times per week when everyone he knew was drinking almost daily. He actually felt bad about it and knew better; that should have been his reference point, not what the others were doing, as he discovered during our session.

Our actions and behaviours are indicative of who we are and what value we place on ourselves. Any behavior that undermines your own value would be a waste of the miracle that you are. That in itself is the worst kind of insult to the Creator.

Where in your life can you take more responsibility? Taking responsibility includes asking for the right kind of help. Do you need that type of guidance?

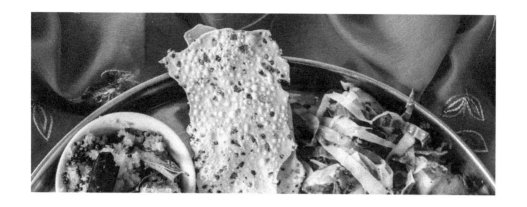

SECTION II

Ayurveda Offers Solutions

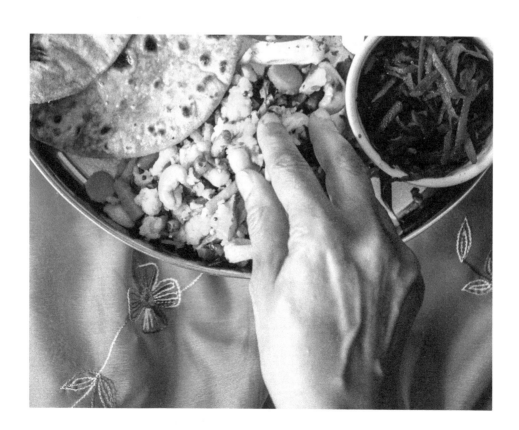

CHAPTER 6

Ayurveda Fills the Gap

Knowing is one thing, but most of us struggle with doing what we know. This path from knowing to doing is riddled with complexity, conflicting information and our own lack of understanding about ourselves. We need clarity and a deeper understanding in order to integrate our knowing into our living. This is where Ayurveda can fill the gap. It provides a system to heal our relationship with food, a system that brings us clarity, common sense and wisdom, a system that provides a bigger context and, is relevant and usable for everyone. Most importantly, Ayurveda provides a system that promises lasting health while ending our battle with food once and for all.

Instead of providing a set of rules to follow and the inducement to forever chase the next best diet, Ayurveda is a dynamic living wisdom that assists us in understanding our lives, ourselves, and our changing needs. It guides us to optimize our health naturally, in alignment with our calling or our purpose. Food is a means to an end. Can we relate to it in a way that creates an inner environment of balance, health and longevity? There is a natural intelligence in food. Can we maintain and harness its intelligence so it supports our health, our purpose and our life? With Ayurveda, we can!

Ayurveda's deep wisdom and understanding is foundational in healing our relationship with food and it empowers us to assess the fad diets and programs that keep us searching for results at the same time as they fail to fulfill the promises they make. Ayurveda is a holistic system that views each individual as a whole and understands that all levels of our existence—physical, emotional and spiritual—are interconnected. Ayurveda starts from the premise that health isn't just about a lack of symptoms, but it's about a balanced mind and body. It recognizes that spirituality and healing are not separate concepts; they are one and the same thing. This is how food becomes our medicine. This system has been here from the beginning of time, it is time-tested, and it is more relevant and needed now than ever before.

THE SCIENCE OF LIFE

The word Ayurveda comes from Sanskrit, and translated into English it means "The Science of Life." It is a vast construct that is more than 6000 years old, and it was cognized by enlightened beings who understood how life works. Under the umbrella of Ayurveda, life works and it makes sense. The interconnectedness of our health to every aspect of our lives provides a matrix that exists everywhere in Nature. Food has been used to heal, to prevent disease and to promote good health and longevity.

Ayurveda's nutritional health system is highly sophisticated, yet it can be greatly simplified, so we can all use this ancient science and wisdom in a meaningful and practical way. It is not a black-and-white science, as it asks that we go beyond the five senses, use our own wisdom and intuition, tune in to the source of our health and longevity, and wake up to our own full potential. It asks us to stop looking for easy answers and develop a deeper understanding within ourselves, one that is fed by our own experiences. It beckons us to tap into the bigger Truth that we already know, use our common sense, and stay true to our nature. There is a magic and mystery to it, just like there is magic and mystery to life which is beyond description but not beyond our experience. When we are talking about common sense, we are talking about using our subtle, yet very powerful senses, and waking up to the Truth that we already know.

We are here to expand, prosper and grow, and to be a light in the world in any way we can; we need more light than we have ever needed before. It is in our true nature to heal and to fulfill our purpose. In a world that is pulling us away from this truth in a very rapid and aggressive way, we need to hold on to it even more fervently, for the sake of the world. But before we run to save the world, we must save ourselves first.

Education goes a long way towards helping people participate in their own healing and in that sense Ayurveda is a participatory medicine. It actively involves the individual. Unlike the passive approach to medicine that does not educate a person, Ayurveda asks people to evolve, grow and deeply connect with their reasons for getting well. In this way, patients feel empowered and can participate in their own health and healing.

Every time I share Ayurveda's wisdom with my clients, it rings true for them. It makes sense to them and there is no questioning it. They feel as if for the very first time they understand what is going on with them, and that relieves the stress and burden they did not even know they were carrying. I wish the same for you, and that this knowledge can be the answer you've been looking for.

For further understanding, it is important to draw a distinction between Ayurvedic medicine and Western medicine. An Ayurvedic practitioner will obtain his or her diagnostic information by feeling a person's pulse on all levels of their body, by touching the skin, by looking at the person's overall appearance, the quality of their speech, how they walk and how they smell; this is much more than merely focusing on the symptoms they are experiencing.

Ayurveda seeks to understand what truly is going on physiologically and psychologically with a patient. Intuition, common sense and the practitioner's level of Consciousness can detect imbalances that no machinery or blood work can ever show. This is a high-touch and highly personal approach, very different from Western medicine, which relies heavily on the results of a blood test or a machine's diagnostics. A wise physician will use both approaches and not limit the patient's treatments to only what aligns with their belief system; he or she will use all methodologies for helping their patients. That is how we bring compassion, care and health back into our so-called health care system. Ayurveda works with Western medicine when that's what the patient needs. The goal is not to collect patients, but to empower them and facilitate the healing process, to bring people to a point where they no longer need the health practitioner.

I am presenting this vast knowledge to you in the simplest way possible. What's presented here is an introduction to the Ayurvedic system to get you thinking and, hopefully, to get you started on your healing journey. This can be the wisdom that can end our turmoil around food and diets. Read this a few times. Let the information sink it. We'll start with some bigger overall concepts that you can begin to think about, and then we will go deeper into each concept so we can apply them on a day-to-day basis.

CONSCIOUSNESS

More commonly understood as awareness, Consciousness is the Source energy out of which awareness arises. Think of it as a field or state of existence. It is an energy that has frequency or vibration and all that we attract into our life is a match for the vibration we internally experience. The same Source energy that created us also created the food we consume. Awareness is not a static phenomenon; it is a continuously expanding state of Consciousness that connects us to our Source. The more aware we are, the better decisions we make. In fact, the quality of our life depends on how aware we are. Although Consciousness is the field out of which awareness arises, I will be using these two terms interchangeably.

Anything we are not aware of is in our *subconscious* mind and it is believed that we live close to 95 percent of our lives subconsciously. This may sound outrageous at first, but the reality is that we have a great deal of untapped potential and life can only get better as we develop more Consciousness.

In order to heal, we must be aware of what needs healing. How we do one thing is how we do everything. How we eat and how we view food is a result of the beliefs about ourselves that we learned during the early years of our lives. Some of those beliefs may not be conducive to how we want to live today. Our professional life, our relationships, and how we live are the result of our subconscious beliefs. As we become more conscious, we can tune into the specific beliefs that are creating habitual patterns in our life. The same beliefs that color our health affect our relationships, our work life and, in fact, all aspects of our life. By becoming more aware, we can decide what beliefs are working against us and use our free will to change those beliefs.

Change is most effective when it is internally driven, rather than externally imposed. When we look to the ever changing information about food that is available to us and try to make changes, these changes are almost always short-lived. With short-term and fragmented changes come short-term and fragmented results. Without understanding what needs changing and why it needs changing, we soon give up. But in the expanded Consciousness, our focus is more on uncovering our potential and becoming whole than it is about just losing a few pounds. This focus pulls us inward, healing us in ways that we never thought possible, and in that larger healing, our relationship with food and everything else begins to shift and heal. This is a more direct and much faster path than hopping from one diet to the next.

Change is a constant in life: our needs, our desires and our inner and outer environments are all dynamic processes of life that require that we be "awake" to them so we can adjust how we live accordingly. Our own experiences are our biggest source of learning and wisdom, and learning to rely on our inner wisdom will empower us in a way that no pill ever can!

WHY DO YOU WANT BETTER HEALTH?

Food is a means to an end. Why do we want better health? Why do we want to lose those few pounds? The answer does not matter as long as you have one. Even if we want to lose weight for vanity reasons, there is something behind that, i.e., it may make us feel more confident, or more beautiful or healthier. There is no wrong answer. So, when we want better health, it is not just for the sake of our health. When we are healthy, we are able to do more, we are able to create our life according to our desires, we can contribute more to our families and our communities; we can excel at everything and, most importantly, we can fulfill our purpose on this planet.

That which can heal us can also destroy us. Our intention and how we use an element is what makes the difference. Alcohol, used medicinally can heal; social media and technology can be used to spread our message and inspire the world. Yet, the same two components can destroy and in fact they have affected millions of people in the most adverse way imaginable. That is why it is important to ask the bigger question so we can really understand what's going on inside of us. This questioning can unravel not only what's going on but the deeply-seated reasons for our challenges.

Solutions are seldom found on the level of the problem; we must get to another level for a bigger and fuller view of the situation. This expands our mind, our thinking and, most importantly, the possibilities available to us. Ayurveda provides that bigger view, as well as a bigger context. We can eat the most potent and miraculous foods, but without understanding our body's changing needs, its ability to break down these foods, the changing external environments and, most importantly, our reasons for eating them, they may not bring the results we expect.

When kale was the miracle food, everyone was adding it into their smoothies, and people were eating and drinking everything kale. It actually created many digestive issues for many of my clients. So, the answer to the question, "Is kale a good food?" is, "It depends on....." And that's how Ayurveda works. It depends on a lot of factors and just because a little bit might be good, a lot can create problems. That's how Ayurveda provides the bigger context, a broader view, under which we can find answers to our smaller questions.

We want food that creates an internal environment of health and vitality so we have the resources to do what we need to do in our life. Food is a means to an end. Ayurveda looks at a bigger and broader view of food and nutrition. Who is eating it? How are they eating it? How often and how much are they eating? What else is going on for this person? It is far from the "one-size-fits-all" approach that we may be more accustomed to in the Western medical world. These are all questions worth asking and this is how food becomes our medicine. Blindly following a fad diet is a far cry from this expanded way of thinking and being.

As I remind my clients, a conscious, healthy life requires that we pay attention and that we care about ourselves enough to think deeper and bigger. Ayurveda is the big umbrella under which all life can function in the most authentic, harmonious and balanced way. Everything affects everything else. It is not about eating or not eating certain foods as all foods (real foods, not processed) are perfect for someone, but nothing is perfect for everyone. And everything can heal us if we use it for that purpose and with that attention. It is for this reason that if we can heal our relationship with food, we can heal our relationship with everything else.

CONNECTION WITH CREATION

We are part of the whole of Creation. Yes, we are! So, we must learn to co-exist with Nature in a way that is harmonious and allows the greater flow of energy within ourselves and that which surrounds us. Nature is everything that is present on this planet. The same energy that created us created the plants and trees, the food, the animals and the environment. As I mentioned earlier, **what we do to**

Nature, we do to ourselves. In the short run, seemingly, we might get away with something…but when our goal is to heal, we are not interested in the narrow vision and what we can get away with in the short run. When you can see yourself in the floating swans, feel yourself in the breeze of the trees and harvest the fruits of the Earth without harming the Earth, you know that there is far more to you than just your physical body. Cruelty towards any part of Creation is cruelty to the whole of Creation and, ultimately, cruelty to us!

Nature's rhythm is also our body's natural rhythm. Synchronizing our natural rhythm to the rhythms of Nature will go a long way towards supporting our own healing. Ordering pizza in the middle of the night is not in harmony with Nature, although we are free to do it. Going against our nature will eventually make us ill. There is a time to sleep, there is a time to wake up, there is a time to eat, there is a time to play, and there is a time to work. We need to eat our biggest meal at lunch time when the sun is at its peak; it is not a coincidence that our digestion is also at its peak during that time. Simply eating our biggest meal at that time will be useful, so it can be properly digested and metabolized, and we can use the energy for the rest of the day.

The five elements (Ether, Air, Fire, Water and Earth) are the building blocks of Creation. The energy, the qualities and the functionality of these building blocks are found everywhere in Nature. The energies and function of these building blocks can also be found in the food we eat. For example, popcorn has mostly the Air element and very little Earth element; pizza, on the other hand, is mostly made of the Earth element. Understanding that is key to knowing what food is good for which person, in what stage of their life, in what season, and in what quantity. In adjusting these variables to get a desired result, we can make food our medicine. We will be discussing in detail how these elements combine to make up our constitution, our imbalances, the different tastes, different seasons, the cycles of our life and our daily cycle. Different combinations of these elements make up our constitution of Vata (Ether and Air), Pitta (Water and Fire), and Kapha (Water and Earth)

ENERGY, QUALITY AND BALANCE

Food is fuel and the quality of the fuel determines the quality of our life. In the conventional sense, we are used to thinking of our quality of life as our lifestyle or our status, our material possessions and the amount of money we have in the bank. Although these are wonderful things to have and enjoy, I am talking about quality of life in terms of our health and well-being. Another word for the energy that food provides to our body is Life Force or Prana. It is not the same as calories. Calories can give you "fuel" to burn, but not vitality or luster. When we eat food that has sufficient calories but is devoid of this Prana, we might miscalibrate our feedback system. When energy is lacking in our food, our body can signal us to continue eating even when sufficient calories have already been consumed. Junk food is a perfect example of this concept. We always want to reach for more. It isn't just because it is stimulating our taste buds; it is because the Prana in the food is missing so we continue to eat more to make up for it.

Pick an apple straight from the tree while it is bathing under the sun and taste it. It tastes like you have tasted the sun, the Earth and the breeze. Now bite on an old apple. The taste will no longer be there. That fresh apple has a higher level of Prana than the old one and it has a pure and fresh energy. It will convey that same energy to our body and mind. Fresh food not only tastes better, it carries a higher level of Prana than old leftover food. Pure foods cause no harm to the environment and therefore the vegetarian diet is considered the purest diet, also called Sattvic diet. (We'll be discussing this, and its companion concepts, in more detail in a later chapter.)

Food nourishes our body, and it also affects our mind and Consciousness as well. Different proportions of the five elements reflect different types of constitution that Ayurveda characterizes as Vata, Pitta and Kapha. Our mental constitution is governed by the three qualities, or fundamental attributes, as well. These three qualities are Sattva, Rajas and Tamas. They affect the quality of Prana, or Life Force, that we experience. And they are equally necessary to maintain our psychological balance. As I mentioned earlier, the five elements are represented in the food we eat and the quality or the energy of that food is governed by the qualities of Sattva, Rajas and Tamas. Our physical and mental health is a function of the balance of the elements and the qualities.

PURITY, MOMENTUM, AND STABILITY

Let's look at the mental qualities first. How we respond to events and circumstances depends on the specific balance of these three qualities (Sattva, Rajas, and Tamas) in our mind. Sattvic qualities imply purity, creativity, clarity, reality, essence and Consciousness. Rajasic qualities provide momentum and energy for us to carry out all the "doing" in our lives. Tamasic qualities help us sustain what we have created and provide stability that supports both the Sattvic and Rajasic qualities. Maintaining a healthy life is about finding a balance amongst these three qualities. It is up to us to become aware when we become too action oriented (Rajas) or too stuck in our ways (Tamas) so we can come into a state characterized by a calm and clear mind (Sattva).

People with predominantly Sattvic qualities are loving, compassionate and pure-minded. They do not anger easily and they look fresh, alert, aware and full of luster; they are recognized for their wisdom, happiness and joy. They are able to maintain mental calm and clarity.

People with predominantly Rajasic qualities tend to be egoistic, ambitious, aggressive, proud, and competitive and they have a tendency to control others. They lead a life marked by sensual enjoyment, pleasure and pain, effort and restlessness, anger and jealousy. They are hard workers and they like prestige, power and position. They become agitated quite suddenly, and they have a fear of failure; they easily become mentally drained. Their task, then, is to soften this quality so they can continue to be compassionate and loving (more Sattvic).

A person with predominantly Tamasic qualities can fall easily into darkness, inertia, heaviness and materialism. This can result in depression, laziness, excessive sleep, eating and drinking. To balance, they need to reduce some of these qualities so they can move towards a more Sattvic life.

The basic nature of our mind is Sattvic, or creative, with just enough Rajas and Tamas to bring our desires to fruition. The balance between these three qualities is vital for health and happiness. A Sattvic mind lends itself to calm, clear and creative thinking that allows the individual to easily resolve problems without too much Rajas and Tamas. Too much Rajas and Tamas distort the natural balance of the mind and have a negative impact on our lives.

There is a connection between how we are eating and how we are acting. Whether a person struggles with depression or committing crimes, we know that food is a big driver of their behaviour. By choosing what we eat, we can choose between Consciousness (Sattva), agitation (Rajas) or inertia (Tamas).

It is important to balance both our physical and our mental constitution. Sattvic food is not necessarily good for all constitutions and imbalances. Some Sattvic food can be too heavy for Vata, too sour for Pitta or too mucus-producing for Kapha. (We'll discuss these ideas in more detail in Chapter 9.)

DIGESTIBILITY AND ENERGY

Our digestive system is like an engine for the vehicle of our human body and life. Digestion is our body's natural process for breaking down the food we eat and transforming it into the fuel or energy we need while getting rid of waste matter. A lack of deeper understanding has led to eating and lifestyle habits that have undermined this innate ability. As mentioned earlier, inflammation is at the root of many illnesses and in our society today we're finding that what we eat, combined with our weakened digestive systems, is causing a lot of inflammation. While ultra-focusing on what we eat, we have under-focused on what we can digest. It is no wonder that in spite of eating the perfect foods, we continue to struggle with digestive issues and ill health.

Our body has an innate ability to heal, if we can only learn to harmonize with its nature and stop getting in its way. So, what we eat is important, but what we digest is far more important for our longevity and vitality.

We are what we digest and what we don't eliminate.

Proper and healthy elimination is part of strong digestion and poor elimination is a sign of poor digestion. Ayurveda expands our digestion beyond our ability to digest food; it also includes our ability to digest our emotions and our experiences. An inability to digest and metabolize our experiences and emotions results in emotional challenges and creates habitual patterns that make life difficult. When our digestion has weakened or we develop food sensitivities, somewhere in there we have not allowed the full expression of our emotions and experiences. I have yet to have one client for whom that has not been true. Even when I am not looking for the psychological factors, they stare me in the face. This puts me in a much better place to be of service to my clients.

Strong digestive power is one of the four pillars of health in Ayurveda. The other three are Sleep, Meditation and Purification. Eating certain foods and eating them at certain times of the day can make us feel bloated, unwell and uncomfortable. This is a sign of a weakened digestive system. There are many serious health issues related to weakened digestion, such as acid reflux, Gastroesophageal Reflux Disease (GERD), food allergies, constipation, lethargy and others. We can take a pill but until we get to the root of the problem, all solutions will be temporary.

While it is wise to eat organic, non-GMO and unprocessed foods, our ability to digest, absorb, assimilate and eliminate the undigested food is far more important, and will give us a deeper insight when making food choices. Our food combinations, the timing of our meals, our internal experiences and the outer environment are some of the factors that affect digestion. Weak digestion is one of the reasons that we can eat the purest and healthiest foods, yet create toxins (which Ayurveda calls Ama) in the body.

There is no magic food or magic pill when it comes to our health and vitality. We are multidimensional beings, and the purpose of food is not to just fill an empty space, but to nourish us on many levels. We are unique in our constitution, tendencies and imbalances, and the one-size-fits-all approach to food just does not work. Moreover, seasonal changes and physiological changes point to the need to look at the whole picture and gain a deeper understanding of how food can be used as a preventive measure, as well as to speed up healing and recovery in the case of an illness.

To sum it all up, the five Ayurvedic concepts or principals we have discussed in this chapter are: Consciousness, Bigger Context, Connection with Creation, Energy, Quality and Balance and Digestibility. Let's look at these concepts in detail in the next chapters.

What are the gaps in your health? Can you find one concept in this chapter that may bridge that gap?

CHAPTER 7

Consciousness and its Role in Healing

As we discussed previously, Consciousness is Source energy and it is the mother of all Creation. Our journey into the physical body begins with Consciousness just like a tree begins with the seed. However, it transcends the human life as we know it and extends beyond the Earth. In other words, it does not end when our human life ends. It has no beginning and no end, and it exists beyond the concept of time and space. It is the source of all our thoughts, and emotions, and our liveliness, and it contains the codes for our energy, information and intelligence. Healing comes from connecting with this Source and disease arises when we are disconnected from it. The challenges that we discussed in the first section of this book dissipate when we become conscious and develop a deep relationship with that part of ourselves that is beyond our body and the mind.

Consciousness is not an intellectual concept; the understanding comes from experiencing it. It is nothing, in the sense that it is devoid of any duality or polarity, and yet it is everything. It is an absolute that contains the energy, information and intelligence that manifests in the physical body. It exists within us as well as outside of us. The nervous system is the seat of our Consciousness. As infants and young kids under age five, we experience the still and the absolute nature of Consciousness and we have a memory of it. Beyond the age of five, we begin to move into the experience of human life and forget our connection with this Source. When we experience it again, it is like coming home to ourselves. We remember that that is who we truly are, Pure Consciousness. Our physical, mental/emotional, energetic, intuitive and spiritual bodies are different expressions of this Consciousness.

HOW DOES CONSCIOUSNESS HEAL?

Experiencing Consciousness is about being in touch with our true Essence. This experience is expansive, whole and blissful and we naturally gravitate towards it. We begin to infuse the experience into our lives. We begin to align our actions, our choices and our lifestyle to what we have experienced. We begin to heal. We move towards acceptance, which spares a lot of our energy that was tied up in worry, control and conflict.

This feeling of wholeness permeates our being. Psychological stress that also caused blockages in the flow of this energy and intelligence begins to dissipate. We now set up the ground for healing and health. What we need to do to heal again becomes clear. We become open to making changes that were not possible before. We tune in to what we need and we find ways to get it. We begin to believe that healing is possible and begin to trust in the bigger picture. We feel part and parcel of this Universe and no longer feel isolated. In deeper parts of us, we begin to believe that all is well. We move towards activities and life styles that promote our health and our growth. Anything else is no longer desirable. It is this shift that allows us to heal and transform our lives.

Any meditation practice that involves transcending beyond the physical aids in experiencing and developing greater Consciousness. Through meditation, we release stress from our nervous system. The mental and emotional imprints on the nervous system begin to loosen their grip, and channels that were blocked begin to open. In this way, we are working at the root cause of illness and we are not just stuck in a limited medical diagnosis.

There is a deep connection between spirituality and healing. To become more conscious is not to control the outcome of our actions; it is rather to co-create with that which is larger. It is to harmonize with our higher Self and let Nature do what is for the highest good. We regain our power when we harmonize with Nature. We heal when we reconnect with the Source out of which all life arises. When we become that tuned in to who we truly are, there is no longer an attachment to a desired outcome, instead we feel okay with whatever happens. We realize that what is in store for us is far more than we could have imagined.

Our individual Consciousness is part of the Unified Field of Consciousness. The laws of Unified Field are the laws of Nature and this is the foundation for Ayurvedic Medicine. It is no longer possible to be Conscious and engage in lifestyles that block our healing.

HOW TO DEVELOP CONSCIOUSNESS

When we talk about living our ultimate Truth, we are talking about the bigger Truth that connects us all. That truth isn't attained by thinking harder; it is only attained by transcending thinking, i.e. not thinking at all.

That is what meditation is! The act of not thinking, not doing, so the truth may surface in the silence and in the non-doing. That Truth is there whether we know it or not. But when we can connect with it via meditation, it is most useful. In that ultimate Truth, our personal truth may surface; the truth of our desires, the truth of our current life, and that holds the key to learning how to heal. So, connecting with the bigger Truth will serve us greatly. The ultimate Truth is that at the core of our existence, we are whole, complete and Pure Consciousness. That is the key to healing our relationship with food, and healing our life.

We are multi-dimensional beings and the only way to restore wholeness is to begin at the Source. Healing happens in our core and not necessarily in the elimination of symptoms. When we heal from within, the symptoms either disappear or no longer get in the way of our happiness.

The deep desire of our being is to feel loved, validated, needed, cherished, and valued and the irony of this is that at our core we are nothing but love. We are worthy and we are on this planet to have a human experience in all that we experience and, ultimately, to rest in the knowing that we are complete and whole at our core.

This is simple but not easy!

Our subconscious is a place of neutrality, in the sense that it does not judge how we fulfill our desires or embody our core beliefs. If the subconscious belief is that "I am unworthy," then our habits and life will continuously try to fill that need by any means possible. Food becomes one of the means.

Until we change our subconscious beliefs, any breakthrough will be temporary and we will find ourselves repeating this pattern over and over again. In order to have a different belief, we must have a different experience; an experience of wholeness. Meditation creates that experience.

Our meditation will feed our emotional hunger in place of the food upon which we've been previously relying to do this.

Patti, a mother of four school-age kids and the wife of a very busy husband came to me one day feeling overwhelmed with all that she had to do. She felt she was continuously on the run and in an emergency mode. She was starting to feel flutters in her chest and she was struggling with anxiety. She worried about the kids and felt guilty if she could not keep up. One of the first things I suggested for her was to learn meditation. She began a meditation practice and came for a follow-up appointment a week later. She felt calm and less intense and was able to accomplish more. She was surprised at the quick results she was obtaining from the meditation. She worried less and finally felt that everything was going to be okay. She felt happy and she looked happy and at peace.

Everyone's experience with meditation will be different and the results are dependent upon the state of one's nervous system and what else is happening in your body and your life. But I have yet to have a client who did not experience benefits from meditation. For many, if not for all my clients, it has been the key to helping them regain their health.

Create some time and space in your life to be still and quiet. Start with five minutes. Notice the effect it has on your life. That is meditation. Learning a technique will help you establish a solid practice. Find a teacher who can teach you this practice.

Pay attention to one area of your life. Are there any patterns that you repeat? What is one pattern that you continuously repeat?

CHAPTER 8

The Bigger Context

Our Consciousness is the subtlest yet the most powerful part of our being and it holds our power to heal. Healing is not just about physical health; it is about the harmonious co-existence of our inner and outer worlds. In the medical field, we think of health as a mere absence of symptoms or of any diagnosable illness. How many of us have no known symptoms yet we just don't feel well? Nothing is wrong, yet something is. That something is our disconnect from our Truth. Our physical symptoms, our mental/emotional turmoil is simply a result of that disconnect. Our symptoms tell us when a disease shows up physically, but that is not where it originates.

Debbie came to me with severe digestive issues. Her doctors suggested surgery, which did not sit well with her as she was barely recovering from a previous surgery for these same issues. After going through the details of the consultation, I asked her what was really going on. That's when she burst into tears and shared with me the story of her marital difficulties. Pressure to make her marriage work at any cost was keeping her quiet and she was outwardly trying to accept the situation. Internally, she was not able to "digest" the state of her marriage, causing the health issues she was experiencing. Giving her some herbs and dietary recommendations without helping her to resolve the underlying cause would not go far. She had never thought about what her expectations and needs were from her marriage. She was denying herself the right to be happy and fulfilled for the sake of keeping the marriage going.

Along with giving Debbie some dietary guidelines, I also guided her to resolve the marital conflict.

In the medical world, the causes of an illness are believed to be physical, hence the endless testing to see what's going on with the physical only. This may be needed, but it isn't the complete picture. At the very best, any psychological issues are referred to a psychologist or a psychiatrist, fragmenting the patient as if their physical health is separate from their psychological health. You may get a little help from pursuing both routes separately, but the whole picture is missed. This creates a huge internal confusion and conflict for the patient and they never really understand what's going on and how to fix it.

We are not a piece of machinery whose parts can be outsourced to different experts to "fix" what's broken. Every part of our being affects every other part and only a holistic view can reveal the real problems.

Rita came to me in the hopes of avoiding surgery for her hip. She was in a wheelchair and had been unable to walk for the previous three years. The lack of movement had caused further tissue deterioration. According to her, she became paralyzed all of a sudden out of the blue. This did not make sense to me as I could not find any physical reasons for her condition. I had picked up from her pulse that there had been a past heartache that had not been resolved. After I ruled everything else out for her condition, I asked her if she had endured a trauma in the past that was not yet healed. And there was. She reported immediately that her inability to walk occurred at the same time as she had felt abandoned by one of her family members. This is the first time that she had connected the trauma to her inability to walk. Now we both knew where the issues were and what needed healing.

The root cause of disease is seldom physical. Healing is about going to those deep root causes and creating shifts there. When we change that one thing in that deep place, changes begin to cascade into every area of our life. Even the smallest shift will have a profound effect, just like a little stir at the bottom of the ocean can create tidal waves.

Healing is built in and healing is what our human journey on this planet is about. Many of us are compelled to go beyond the physical when struck with a terminal illness, a tragedy or just one of life's challenges. This innate healing is your Truth, the wholeness that is trying to find you.

Spirituality is about connecting with your spirit, as it knows the truth, and healing is the experience or result of that connection. All healing in that regard is spiritual.

In the world of fixing, improving and navigating the web of societal conditioning, spiritual healing is a breath of fresh air awakening us to the knowing that we are whole, and are at the perfect place and time in our lives. It is in this place that the process becomes more of Self-discovery than of self-improvement. This is where we know that we can heal from anything and overcome any obstacles that get in our way. We can always take a pill! And at times, it may be necessary for a short while so we can start to think straight. But if we really want to heal at every level of our existence, then we must dig deeper, ask the bigger questions and develop a bigger context for our health.

"Why do you think you are having the health issues that you are having?" Asking this question to my clients takes them beyond the symptoms and allows their life story to emerge. They often begin to see how the same story is playing out in other areas of their life, such as their work and their relationships. Simply the willingness to look beyond the physical symptoms raises the level of our awareness and we begin to see a bigger picture than we had before. That in itself is empowering and begins the healing process at the level of our awareness.

UNRESOLVED STORIES AND DISEASE

More times than not, a disease is about our unresolved story. The only way to resolve or to heal the story is to go into the experience of it. What we experience at the cellular level will continuously repeat in other areas of our life and in our illness, until it is resolved. The only way to heal that experience is first to allow it and open our heart to it as it is very much a part of who we are. And then we may ask the bigger question. What may I learn from this experience? What's the lesson? This is where we do the work, dig a little deeper and learn and heal what we need to heal. Our beliefs change, our habits line up and our body begins to heal.

When we realize that we have the power to change our story, we begin to heal.

This work isn't easy. It requires a certain kind of stamina, but it is definitely easier than living with an illness. You may experience resistance in all kind of different ways, rationalizing the situation away or pretending that all is okay, when it isn't. Fear shows up in all kinds of distorted ways. This is where you need expert guidance to help you through. Healing is an organic process. We can't will it or force it to occur. We allow it and stay present to it. That is healing! It has its own timing, and we can facilitate it by getting out of the way.

These are the ancient teachings and the wisdom. We can heal from anything if we use it for that purpose and with that intention. Healing requires that we be willing to take a deep dive within and can stay the course. **Healing is chosen, while illness happens by default.** You can heal from anything and overcome the blocks that show up in the process. I believe that! In order for you to heal, you must believe that, too. We have the power to heal ourselves.

Annie came to me wanting to get off her medication for colitis. In spite of doing everything right, she felt her body had abandoned her. As we continued to work deeper, abandonment was the recurring theme in her life and it started with the passing of one of her parents. Since then she tried hard to hold on to the people in her life out of fear of being abandoned. That was the unresolved issue that had manifested as colitis. It was a big relief for her to discover this and to connect the physical to her emotions. Now we both knew where she needed help.

What's unresolved in your life? Something always is, as our lives are a work-in-progress. When we are conscious of it, we see the unresolved as it is, rather than giving it more power than it deserves. When we give it more power, that's when it can manifest physically.

CHAPTER 9

Our Connection with Creation

We are each a part of the whole of Creation. That which created us created everything around us. The five elements, Ether, Air, Fire, Water and Earth, are the building blocks of Creation. They are categorized from the subtle, light and intangible to the heavy, dense and gross, with Ether being the subtlest and Earth being the densest element. Everything in Creation can be understood in relation to these five elements, in a way that is similar to how light can be separated into the seven colors of the rainbow. Creation is a cyclical and dynamic process, continuously changing and flowing. Something is being created and something is being destroyed all the time to maintain balance.

These elements are fluid forces that work with one another to create cycles of the seasons, of day and night, of our life and our internal cycles. We know these elements in their raw form as space, breeze, sun, water and the earth beneath our feet. The way to understand these elements is to understand their qualities and their function, and to learn how they operate in everything living. These elements work interdependently, each affecting the other; so, more than just science, we need deep wisdom and intuition to keep them all balanced. Each element has its desirable and not-so-desirable qualities. When we talk about bringing balance into our life and our health, we want to harness the most desirable qualities of these elements and minimize their undesirable qualities.

The variety of foods, of body and personality types, of animals, and all the variety in plants and trees, can be understood in terms of which element is most predominant. Each element combines with another element for its most desirable expression, for example, Earth and Water join together to make mud—the stuff that holds our homes and our bodies together (Kapha). Fire combines with a little bit of Water (so it does not burn and dry things up) to heat things like our digestive fire (Pitta). Air and Space together can move things, such as pollen in the spring or food in our body (Vata).

Vata, Pitta and Kapha, can also be viewed as forces that are continuously destroying (Vata), organizing (Pitta) and Generating (Kapha) to maintain balance. The combination of these elements is what gives rise to our constitution and our imbalances. Imbalances are called Dosha in Sanskrit. Literally translated, Dosha means "that which is spoiled," as any of the three forces can be out of balance. To heal is to balance these forces in our life. Each one of us has a unique body and personality type, and we need and desire different things, and for that reason we each need a unique approach to food and our diet. We need all five elements in our food, in our life and in our body to live a balanced life. Let's look at each element separately to understand them better.

ETHER OR SPACE

The nature of this element is expansive, open, subtle and soft. The Ether element is considered to be the first expression of Consciousness into Creation. This element is formless and it is the subtlest of all the elements. It provides space for all the other elements to function so it takes on the qualities of the other elements that are operating within it. This element is all around us; without Space, we can't exist. We clearly experience this element at the beach or the park where there is a lot of open space.

Ether is also represented by the channels or spaces in our body where all our bodily functions take place. Our spirit is of the Ether element and many cultures have practices of fasting to connect with that element via prayer or meditation. When we are fasting, we are not taking in other elements via our food, and therefore we are creating more Space. Having too much of this element can make us feel spacy and depleted, and having too little can make us feel rigid or stuck. As mentioned earlier, each element works with another elements for its expression. Space combines with Air to give rise to Vata, which is a destroying force. It moves or separates and destroys the previous cycles in our body, in Nature and in life.

AIR

The nature of this element is irregular, mobile, expansive, dry, light, rough, cold and subtle. This is the next level in the expression of Consciousness, and this is the point where Consciousness takes a particular direction. This element is formless but it's less subtle than the Ether element. The most important function of this element is movement. It combines with Space for its best expression. Spreading of pollen and a soft breeze are desirable functions of this element but in excess they give rise to tornadoes that create destruction. When in excess, this element can be fierce and destructive.

Air element is responsible for all the movements in our body. The movement of our breath, our blood circulation, the movement of food, and all communications are a function of this element. Air is responsible for the electric energy in our nervous system, the movement of all tissues, the functioning of our hearing, and speaking and our sense of touch. Having too much Air can make us feel bloated and gassy and having too little can make us feel stuffy and stuck. But we need just the right amount to feel balanced.

Popcorn, crackers and leafy greens are of predominantly Air element. Having too much of these foods, for a person who is predominantly made up of this element (Vata dosha) and especially in the winter months (which is Vata season, as discussed below) can cause depletion, as Air is destructive when present in excess.

FIRE

This element is hot, sharp, light, dry and dynamic. The most important function of this element is to transform and it is needed for Consciousness to express itself into form. This element provides dynamism, heat and power. It combines with the next element, Water, for its best expression and is the organizing power of Creation. Too little sun can dampen everything and too much can burn. Without the sun, most plants can't grow and produce. Again, we need just the right amount for its balanced function. For example, we need just the right amount of heat to cook our food.

This element is responsible for the digestive fire in the body. It is needed to transform and metabolize our food into the energy we need. Weakened digestion leads to many illnesses, so balancing this element in our body can be the single most important and health-promoting action we can take. Ayurveda always looks at the whole picture; just as enough Fire is needed to transform our food; it is also needed to transform our emotions into intelligence, and to transform our experiences into wisdom. It is responsible for maintaining optimal body temperature, and the absorption and assimilation of food, as well as for the transformative power of the liver.

We need some Fire in the foods we eat to transform them into energy and we add that by spices, not just hot, pungent spices, but also many other spices and herbs that can add a little heat to the food to make it easier to digest. Hot, spicy food has a predominance of Fire element in it, and so does a fiery temperament. The same heat that can keep us warm during the winter months can, in excess, inflame our body. Our body is always trying to achieve homeostasis, a point of balance. When we eat, we want to eat in a balanced way. Someone with a fiery personality (Pitta dosha) will become more fiery by eating hot and spicy foods (Pitta foods), especially in the summer months (Pitta season), so eating cooling foods is needed to balance the emotions.

Chili peppers, ginger, cinnamon, cumin, black pepper are some examples of foods with Fire predominance.

WATER

The nature of this element is fluid, cold, dull, soft, slimy or oily, and mobile. Fire transforms Consciousness into this next level of its expression, the first expression with form. The most important function of this element is nurturance and cohesion, to hold things together and in that sense its function can be compared to a mother that nurtures the family and holds it together. No processes in the body can take place without Water. Its most important function is transportation. It is the carrier or the medium through which all processes take place. Water takes on the qualities of the other elements that it combines with. As it combines with Fire, it works to balance the Fire so it does not get too hot. When combined with Earth, it becomes mud that holds things together.

Too much of this element can cause floods and too little can create drought. Again, we need just the right amount for its balanced function. Balance is not a static point; it is a dynamic process where these elements are always working to move toward that state over time.

Water manifests as the plasma and lymph systems in our body that bring nutrients to our cells and carry toxins away from the cells. It governs our sense of taste and our reproductive function. Our body is estimated to be 60-70% water. This element nurtures the cells, detoxifies our organs and connects the whole body together.

Celery, cucumber, and melons are good examples of foods with a predominance of this element. Carbohydrates also fit this category due to their ability to glue things together, hence the need for carbohydrates and fats. Too much can cause gluten sensitivity, which is actually a way for us to reduce the amount of carbs we consume. This is how balance is built into the body, and is attained.

EARTH

The nature of this element is heavy, dull, constant, dense and gross. This is where Consciousness fully takes form and becomes substance. It is this element that holds and cradles everything together, providing support, energy, and structure. Too much of this element can result in stagnation and rigidity and too little results in instability. Creation is always working to find balance so just the right amount of this element needs to be present for the other elements to express themselves fully as well.

The Earth element in our body creates immunity, strength, and stability, and manifests as bones, muscles, cartilage, nails, hair, teeth and skin. It combines with the element Water for its best expression. Too much of this element can manifest as "couch potato syndrome," lethargy, a tendency to being overweight, obese and, on the psychological side, hoarding and holding on to things, old grudges and emotions.

Foods with Earth element predominance are meats, root vegetables, cheeses and sweets, protein and minerals. We need a sufficient amount of these to sustain our muscles, strength and our immunity. Now let's discuss how these five elements are expressed in our body, our mind, in seasons, in cycles of the day and night, in different tastes, and in foods.

ELEMENTS IN OUR BODY AND OUR MIND

As mentioned earlier, each element combines with another element to give rise to the three forces that can be seen and experienced everywhere in our world. Ether and Air combine to give rise to Vata. Water and Fire combine to give rise to Pitta. Water and Earth combine to give rise to Kapha.

Vata, Pitta and Kapha are the Generating, Organizing and Destroying forces in our body and our being and they are always working to bring balance within us. (We can abbreviate them as GOD). And, while we each have all of these forces within us, one tends to predominate. When we refer to these forces at work in the body they are called Constitutions, or "Dosha" in Sanskrit. (Although "Dosha" is used to describe an imbalance, the word is used interchangeably with "constitution.")

VATA CONSTITUTION

Ether and Air combine to create a Vata constitution and those blessed with this dosha may be unusually short or unusually tall but they will have a small frame, and are always very thin. They tend to be vivacious, talkative, creative and enthusiastic but may have hard time staying on task and being focused; they may fidget. Please note that the most desirable and the most undesirable qualities of any dosha can be found within the same person, and most of us are trying to get to a "balanced" state where the undesirable qualities of Vata—such as too much talking, a tendency towards hyperactivity, and an inability to focus—are minimized. Too much of the undesirable qualities of this dosha can result in insomnia, anxiety, fear, constipation, bloating, arthritis, food sensitivities and allergies, and depletion, among other issues. Someone with a balanced Vata demonstrates more of the desirable qualities of Vata, which are creativity, enthusiasm, softness and balanced movement.

Vata governs the other doshas so it is always a good idea to keep this dosha in balance.

Woody Allen is a perfect example of someone with Vata constitution. A chipmunk is another one. (Every time I see one, I call it a Vata-deranged creature.)

Due to their creative nature, those with Vata constitution, tend to hop from project to project continuously looking for stimulation. Like their predominant elements, Ether and Air, they don't like routines, schedules or discipline. They want to do whatever they want, whenever, which makes them feel easily overwhelmed. This leads to worry, anxiety and other challenges. The natural tendency for Vata is to enjoy things and foods that are close to their nature. They love running, and enjoy Vata foods such as salads, crackers, cold and raw foods, soft drinks, and popcorn, and they tend to eat on the run. **Like increases like** and too much of these foods create a Vata imbalance with some or all of the issues mentioned previously.

Understanding our constitution helps us understand our nature and what's needed to get back to balance. Our deeper understanding and our awareness can help lead us back to balance. In spite of the natural tendency of Vata people to eat lightly and flit from one activity to another, they need routine, discipline and warm, cooked, and oily foods in order to get back into balance. For them to enjoy their free and creative nature, they need an anchor, boundaries and discipline in their lives. Otherwise, they will end up expressing their most undesirable qualities. Foods that pacify Vata are discussed below.

Sharon came to me experiencing high anxiety and fear. She loved being physically active and enjoyed dancing and running. She ate healthily, or so she thought: lots of salads were always on her menu. She had recently lost her husband and she had become more fearful of being alone. Sharon was very thin and she had a small build (the hallmarks of a Vata constitution). With her activities and eating (running and dancing are Vata activities, and salads are Vata foods) she was creating an imbalance that created more fear and anxiety in the wake of her husband passing away. I recommended that she stop running and enroll in Yoga. I also recommended that she eat more cooked, warm and oily foods. She also learned meditation. Vata people need lots of security, boundaries and love. I suggested that she join some meet-up groups to meet people. She followed all of my recommendations diligently (this is not always the case with my clients!). At one of her appointments, she asked if it was okay that she was feeling so happy and that anxiety was nowhere to be found. That turned out to be her last appointment. She loved Yoga so much that she is now teaching it.

PITTA CONSTITUTION

Those with Pitta constitution have a medium build and are muscular and athletic. Fire and Water predominate in their constitutions. When in balance, these types are sharp, generous, social, focused and they have big personalities. They are organized, decisive, and they see things clearly, but they can be intense and they may have sharp tempers. Another characterstic that stands out for Pitta people is that they often have red hair and skin.

Tom Cruise is a good example of someone with Pitta constitution. In the animal kingdom, the tiger fits the bill.

A balanced Pitta is sharp, focused, generous, social, and calm, and this is the ideal expression of who they are.

Due to their fiery nature, Pitta people mean business. Stay out of their way when their mind is set on something. They don't like to waste time. They are sharp as a razor and a force to be reckoned with. When things don't go their way, they can become angry and irritated. They like to be in charge of everything. They have an intense appetite. They naturally enjoy hot spicy foods, meat and alcohol, tomatoes, garlic and onions. They live large. Eating Pitta foods and leaning into their personalities creates more Pitta and leads to Pitta imbalance which may manifest as psoriasis, skin conditions, hypertension, and migraine headaches.

To recreate balance, those with Pitta constitution need to stop and smell the roses. A walk in the cool moonlight and swimming are some cooling activities that can bring them balance. Another way is by cutting down on hot spicy foods and increasing cooling bitter foods. Keep reading to find out which foods are pacifying for a Pitta constitution.

Paul, who had a Pitta constitution, came to me due to arthritis that was showing up in his hands. His face and skin were red, as though inflamed. When I asked about his diet, he excitingly informed me how much he loved hot and spicy foods. In fact, he was very proud of his collection of different chili sauces. I was not surprised when he told me he loves grapefruit, tomatoes, garlic and onions. These are all Pitta foods and they were helping him create a Pitta imbalance (inflammation in his hands.) And, yes, he loved people, socializing and alcohol. Although, this was a challenge, the way for him to balance was to reduce his consumption of Pitta foods, which would reduce the inflammation he was experiencing, while increasing his consumption of cooling foods—such as bitter greens—and adding anti-inflammatory spices like turmeric to help him get his pain under control.

KAPHA CONSTITUTION

With the predominance of Water and Earth elements, those with Kapha constitution have a large build and a large frame; they are heavy and soft. They like to have a plan and they love routine. They are very reliable and have a good, gentle nature. When in balance, they are sweet, jovial, and kind, and they have a teddy bear-type personality. When out of balance, they can become couch potatoes, lethargic, and obese.

Santa Claus is a good example of Kapha, and in the animal kingdom, we see Kapha in the elephant.

A balanced Kapha is very stable, consistent and reliable; they are generous and kind, and they have soft personalities.

Kapha people like to collect things and they like to have a lot. They like luxury and excessive buying, and they don't engage in anything creative. They enjoy sedentary activities and love to sit, watch movies, and talk. They love heavy foods, such as pizza, cheese, ice cream, meat products, and sweets. They often overeat. This leads to Kapha imbalance and can manifest as couch potato syndrome, obesity, diabetes, depression and heart conditions, to name a few.

In order to balance, those with Kapha constitution should incorporate lighter foods (Vata foods) such as leafy greens, salads and light soups, and they should minimize heavy foods, such as dairy and meat products. Exercise for them is a must, as they tend to be sedentary. We'll look at Kapha balancing foods later.

Gail came to me due to her inability to lose weight. She was about 200 pounds overweight, and she was a great, passionate cook. She loved to eat and party. The weight gain had occurred over the years as a result of too much eating, socializing and living large. The more weight she gained, the harder it became to move around and the less she wanted to move. Although she had originally had a Pitta constitution and imbalance, she ignored it for too long and thus created a Kapha imbalance. As passionate as she was, it became a real struggle for her to move, even when she knew she had to. Moving or working out was painful, and therefore she did not want to do it. This is why it is so important to stay in balance: when an imbalance is ignored for too long, it can become a deeply-ingrained problem, both mentally and physically.

Gail and I had to take small steps to change her mindset and I had to become strict with her, as that is what she needed at this point in order to make a shift. Gale is working hard to change her situation, even though it is challenging for her.

It is important to understand that these three forces, Vata, Pitta and Kapha are continuously working in our body to create homeostasis and we need all three of them. In general, the constitution of an individual and their imbalances tend to be the same, but this is not necessarily true. For example, those with Vata constitution tend to have a Vata imbalance, those with Pitta constitution tend to have a Pitta imbalance and those with Kapha constitution tend to have a Kapha imbalance. But Vata individuals can equally create a Pitta or a Kapha imbalance. Similarly, Pitta people can create a Vata or a Kapha imbalance, and those with Kapha constitution can create a Vata or Pitta imbalance. To determine a person's constitution and imbalance, we look at their physical body, its functions, and their psychological nature.

Take a look at the chart on the following page and fill it out to discover your constitution and a possible current imbalance.

DISCOVERING YOUR CONSTITUTION AND IMBALANCE

VATA	PITTA	KAPHA
☐ Small frame and thin	☐ Medium frame and athletic build	☐ Large frame and big build
☐ Small ankle and wrist bones	☐ Medium ankle and wrist bones	☐ Large ankle and wrist bones
☐ Thin face	☐ Square or medium face	☐ Large or round face
☐ Small, and active, dark eyes	☐ Medium and penetrating eyes	☐ Large eyes with thick eyelashes
☐ Thin, dark and rough hair	☐ Light, blond or red, fine, oily hair	☐ Thick wavy hair, dark or light
☐ Dry and thin skin	☐ Skin is oily and a little heavier	☐ Thick and moist skin
☐ Cold hands and feet	☐ Always warm	☐ Sweats easily
☐ Brittle nails	☐ Flexible and strong nails	☐ Strong thick nails
☐ Has a hard time gaining weight	☐ Can gain/lose weight easily at will	☐ Gains weight easily, has a hard time losing it
☐ Appetite is variable	☐ Voracious appetite	☐ Enjoys eating, finds it hard to stop and can easily skip meals
☐ Likes to snack, nibble	☐ Likes high protein meals	☐ Loves fatty, heavy, starchy foods
☐ Food sensitivities	☐ Can eat anything	☐ Sluggish digestion
☐ Variable thirst	☐ Usually thirsty	☐ Rarely thirsty
☐ Tends towards constipation	☐ Tends towards a loose stool	☐ Soft, regular bowel movements
☐ Light, restless sleep	☐ Needs only 6 hours of sleep	☐ Can sleep all day
☐ Prefers warm climate, sunshine	☐ Prefers cool and airy places	☐ Likes all climates except humid ones
☐ Dislikes routine	☐ Likes routine and being in charge	☐ Likes routine
☐ Creative thinker	☐ A leader and a visionary	☐ Good at organizing
☐ Likes to be physically active	☐ Likes physical activities, especially competitive ones	☐ Loves sedentary activities
☐ Learns quickly & forgets quickly	☐ Analytical mind	☐ Rarely forgets, good memory
☐ Changes mind easily	☐ Has strong opinions	☐ Changes opinions slowly
☐ Tends toward fear/anxiety when stressed	☐ Tends toward frustration/anger when stressed	☐ Tends to avoid difficult situations
☐ Changeable mood and ideas	☐ Likes to express ideas and feelings	☐ Steady, reliable, slow to change
☐ Mind tends to race	☐ Very focused with a sharp mind	☐ Calm mind
☐ Enthusiastic but unfocused	☐ Goal oriented and has a sharp focus	☐ Easy-going and needs motivation
____ **Number of Checks**	____ **Number of Checks**	____ **Number of Checks**

The column with the most checks is usually your primary constitution. If you have an equal number of checks in two or all three columns, then you are bi-doshic such as vata-pitta, or pitta-vata, vata-kapha or pitta-kapha etc. Or you could be tri-doshic.
If you checked some aspects under a column that are different from your constitution as a whole, then you could have that imbalance. For example, if your primary dosha is vata, as that's what has the most checks, but if you also checked two-three issues under the pitta or kapha column, especially the psychological and physical functions, then you could have either a pitta or a kapha imbalance.

ELEMENTS IN THE SEASONS

The seasons are a result of changes in Nature that in turn create changes in our body and its needs. This means we need to change what we eat in the changing seasons. Please note that the seasons listed below are for people in Northern Hemisphere. You may need to adjust if you live in other parts of the world.

VATA SEASON

Vata season is late fall and early winter. The weather turns cold, the wind blows, and the earth becomes dry, hard, cold and rough. With the unpredictable and irregular nature of Vata season, it is best to minimize Vata foods such as cold and raw foods as that would create more of the Vata imbalance. **In order to bring balance, we introduce foods of the opposite qualities.** To stay balanced in the Vata season, it is best to favor warm, cooked and oily foods such as stews, soups, cooked root vegetables, and hot beverages, and eat sufficient quantities of them. The colder weather can sometimes make people want to stay inside and be more sedentary than in other seasons. It is important that we don't become too sedentary, and we must maintain our regular exercise routines. Since Vata tends to be erratic and irregular, it is important to maintain a regular schedule of eating, sleeping and exercising in order to balance Vata.

When we over-indulge during the winter months on sweets or holiday treats, we can create a Kapha imbalance, i.e. gain weight. It is very common during this time for people to gain weight. It's okay to gain a little weight gain if you have a small build, but too much can be problematic. So, eat enough to maintain your balance but don't go overboard. One way to make sure of that is to undertake regular rigorous exercise at least three or four times a week. Exercise is important all the time, but more so in the Vata season due to our tendency to go "dormant" and eat more.

KAPHA SEASON

Kapha season is from late winter to early spring. The snow melts (if there is snow where you live), sap rises, the ground becomes muddy and the trees blossom. Kapha season is characterized by heavy, dense, wet, gooey, stable, and cool qualities. Much like Nature, this is the time when our body will try to get rid of accumulated Kapha over the winter months in order to reach balance. We might experience this as colds, sinus discomfort or allergies, and we might feel lethargic and heavy. In order to help our body get rid of this excess Kapha, we need to switch up our diet. Eating foods that are lighter, drier and pungent (as discussed more in the tastes section of this chapter) will allow us to move all that winter-derived Kapha out of our body. As soon as they are available, eat the first bounty of the season: sprouts, berries, dandelions and other spring greens, which naturally support this time of cleansing. Avoiding processed food, sugars and caffeine is a great way to help our body naturally detoxify. Eating less fat and animal products, heavy and sweet foods is also recommended.

PITTA SEASON

Pitta season is from mid-June to mid-September—the summer months. We need to stay cool during these months. Summer's bounty offers plenty of ways to keep cool: cucumbers, mint, summer squash, zucchini, melons, sweet, juicy fruits, berries, coconut water and mangoes. Our digestion slows down in the summer to compensate for the external heat. To keep our digestion strong, it is best not to overindulge in ice cold beverages and ice-cream, as they reduce the efficiency of our digestive system (more about that in our chapter on digestion). While a little of these foods can help us stay cool, too much can dampen our digestive power, making the system work harder and, in turn, create more heat. Staying cool and light is the way to maintain balance in this season.

ELEMENTS IN THE TIMES OF DAY AND NIGHT

Just as different elements predominate in different seasons, different elements are predominant at different times of the day and night.

VATA TIME

Air and Ether are predominant in the environment during Vata Time and it occurs from 2:00-6:00 a.m. and 2:00-6:00 p.m. The morning hours represent an auspicious time to meditate and pray and to connect with our spirit or our guides. The Vata energy is creative energy, making the mid-afternoon hours a perfect time for creative work such as writing and other projects.

KAPHA TIME

The elements Water and Earth are predominant during Kapha time and it occurs between 6:00-10:00 a.m. and 6:00-10:00 p.m. Kapha energy is heavy and stable, so exercising during the morning Kapha time is a valuable antidote for the heaviness of that time of day. But going with the flow of this energy in the evening hours of Kapha time helps us slow down, unwind, and relax our nervous system so we can get ready for sleep. Eating a lighter meal in the evening is recommended, as that's when our digestion and metabolism are slower. Heavy meals consumed in the evening Kapha time can create more toxicity in the body.

PITTA TIME

Fire and Water are predominant in the environment during Pitta Time, between 10:00 p.m.-2:00 a.m. and 10:00 a.m.-2:00 p.m. Pitta energy is sharp, intense and hot. It's best to eat our largest meal during the day at this time, because our digestive power is intense and at its peak. During the overnight Pitta hours, our digestive Fire turns inward "cleaning" the GI track, and allowing us to sleep deeply so we may wake up refreshed and recharged. It is recommended that we retire for bed before 10:00 p.m. so we don't risk the return of our hunger and the midnight snack attack that might result. Falling asleep before Pitta time allows our digestion to turn inward and do all the processing it needs to do to help us awaken refreshed and renewed the next day.

Understanding the cycles of day and night can help us create a simple daily routine which is very balancing for Vata. The routine can incorporate waking up just a little before 6:00 a.m. and being in bed just a little before 10:00 p.m. Exercising in the morning and slowing down in the evening allows us to harness the Kapha energy appropriately and efficiently. Eating a light, warm, cooked breakfast, with a big meal during the mid-day Pitta time, and a lighter meal in the evening, will help us harmonize with these elements in the environment and create balance for ourselves.

ELEMENTS IN THE CYCLES OF OUR LIFE

From birth to puberty, we are in Kapha time (the spring of our lives) of our lives. From puberty to 60 is Pitta time (the summer of our lives) and after 60 is Vata time (the winter of our lives). When we are young, we need lots of food and protein to build our body. In the middle of our lives, we need to eat to sustain our energy and vitality. And, in our older years, we can do with lighter foods, generally speaking. There are always exceptions and other factors that determine how we eat, such as our ability to digest, our body weight, our constitution, and our imbalances.

ELEMENTS IN THE TASTES

Our food choices are greatly influenced by the tastes we like. Although this is a good indicator of which tastes to include in our diet, without understanding the effects of those tastes on our body, we can overdo it on some tastes, and not have enough of others. This creates an imbalance in our physiology and results in cravings which can help us tune into the tastes that may be missing in our meals. The solution, however, may not be as simple as just adding those tastes to our meals. For example, when we feel down or tired, we may crave the Sweet taste. As much as that taste can provide a quick pick-me-up, overdoing it can also lead to more fatigue. Moreover, the source of the Sweet taste matters: cookies or dates? The best solution is to figure out what's causing our fatigue and to include the taste we need in our meals—preferably via fresh foods, rather than treats. Similarly, a craving for coffee may indicate that the Bitter taste is missing in our meals. Bitter taste makes us feel light and energetic. The solution is to add Bitter taste via bitter greens in our diet, rather than going overboard on coffee.

A deeper understanding of the tastes is needed. Different tastes have different digestive and post-digestive effects on our bodies. A balanced meal includes six different tastes altogether: Sweet, Salty, Sour, Pungent, Astringent and Bitter. Different tastes stimulate the secretion of different enzymes for digestion, so our system can work optimally and ultimately satisfy our body's need for all the tastes. This curbs cravings!

Our sense of taste can give us a guide map to proper nutrition, provided we understand a little more about the different tastes and their effect on our body and our emotions. There is intelligence behind each taste, and our cravings can give us deep insight into what's going on with our body and what's taking place emotionally. Our taste buds identify tastes, of course, but they also unlock the nutritive value of food and provide an initial spark for the digestive process.

Each of the six different tastes communicates intelligence to our body, providing coded information to our nervous systems that relates to a meal's nutritional content. If we eat foods that correspond to each of these tastes throughout the day, our meals will provide diverse nourishment that leaves us feeling satiated. If we do not have all six tastes in our diet, our brain receives signals calling for more food, because our body's nutritional needs have not been satisfied. So, we keep eating, and we take in too many calories, even though we remain undernourished.

In a perfect world, all six tastes are accounted for at every meal. But let's examine one taste at a time to see how we can improve our health through the food we eat.

SWEET TASTE

Sweet taste is composed of the elements Earth and Water. The qualities of this taste are heavy, moist, consolidating, soothing and cooling, and these are the qualities that are imparted to our body and mind via this taste. Like its constituent elements, Sweet is a stabilizing taste; it can increase lubrication, tone areas of deficiency and calm the nerves. Because of its consolidating quality, for many, Sweet taste is a nice way to finish off a meal.

Sweet taste is the most pleasurable taste and hence the reason for its overconsumption. It is also considered a celebratory taste. It is customary to have it at weddings, birthdays and other special occasions by way of cakes and other sweet treats. We can also overdo it on Sweet taste by overconsuming fruits such as mangoes, oranges, pineapple, and even apples. This is the taste that is most responsible for many health problems, such as weight gain, inflammation, and diabetes, to name a few. On the other hand, having too little of this taste can be depleting to our bodies, and can cause irritation.

The reality is that people rarely have too little Sweet taste in their diet; it is mostly consumed to excess. Sugary treats are now available all the time and enjoying a desert after a meal has become more common. Not only that, but refined sugar in various forms is in all the processed foods that are readily available to soothe our discomforts and sedate us; hence the reason it is so addictive. Even if we are not deliberately adding Sweet taste to our meals, simply chewing food extracts the sweetness from it, and that's the ideal way to experience Sweet taste in our meals.

Not too much and not too little is the Ayurvedic way. So, having a cookie or ice-cream once in a while is fine, but having them after every meal would be too much. You also want to allow a little gap after a meal, of at least 30 minutes, so your food can be digested before loading your system with sugar. This prevents fermentation of your undigested food and the resulting toxicity.

Sweet taste can be very grounding for Vata people, as its elements of Earth and Water are balancing to the elements predominant in those with Vata constitution (Ether and Air). Sweet taste can be cooling for Pitta people but for Kapha people, it adds more of the same elements (Earth and Water) that can lead to too much Kapha. This is toxic to the physiology and promotes the already-problematic sedentary lifestyle among Kapha people.

The healthiest way to add Sweet taste to our meals is by enjoying sweet-tasting vegetables such as carrots, beets, sweet potato, squashes and peas. Other foods with Sweet taste include dairy products, sweet juicy fruits, nuts, seeds, grains, legumes, meat and eggs. Many foods have a natural sweetness to them, and chewing them well extracts the Sweet taste, which is one of the reasons grandma told us to chew our food well.

Sweet taste is balancing in the winter months (Vata Season) and should be avoided in the spring time (Kapha Season) as our bodies naturally seek to detoxify from the overconsumption of Sweet taste during the winter months Enjoying the fresh juicy sweet fruits in the summer months (Pitta Season) is a great way to include the Sweet taste and to balance the heat.

Overconsumption of Sweet taste can indicate a desire or need for love, comfort and nurturance. *A client who had a death in the family began baking cupcakes and enjoying them, as this was her way of nurturing herself.* We can find other ways for self-love and nurturance so we don't overdo the Sweet taste. Self-massage with oil, prayer and meditation, eating well, and getting enough sleep are some of the ways to take care of yourself in challenging times. Ultimately, all tastes merge into the taste of sweetness if we allow ourselves to fully enjoy our meals.

Cutting out refined sugar completely from your diet can be the one single thing you can do to move towards bettering your health. Many of my clients have lost weight and reduced the inflammation-led incidences of aches and pains in their body as a result of this one single change.

SALTY TASTE

Salty taste is composed of the elements Fire and Water. The qualities of this taste are hot, heavy and moist. Its heating quality stimulates digestion and improves the taste of foods. Like Sweet taste, Salty taste tends to be somewhat moist and heavy, not as much as Sweet taste, and yet a little more than Sour taste. It stimulates water retention, and is initially warming, but its long-term action is more moistening and grounding and not very warming.

Excessive use of this taste creates more intensity and stimulation, which can be addictive. Examples are potato chips or corn chips; once you begin eating them, it is often difficult to stop. Just like the Sweet taste, overconsumption of Salty taste is common and problematic. The Salty taste can be as addictive as Sweet taste. Overuse can be heating to our body, causing inflammation and irritation to the mucus lining of the stomach, which creates burning after eating. Too little Salty taste can be drying.

Salty taste is a balancing taste for those with Vata constitution (Ether and Air) and in excess can imbalance Pitta (Fire and Water) and Kapha (Earth and Water). Reducing salt consumption in spring and summer is a great way to balance our body in these seasons, especially for those with Pitta (Water and Fire) and Kapha (Water and Earth) constitution.

It's best to add a little bit more salt to your meals, rather than eating salty snacks. Common Salty foods include salt, sea or rock salt, and sea vegetables like seaweed, kelp, salted nuts and chips.

Salt cravings may point out to the need to find passion or some zing in your life.

SOUR TASTE

Sour taste is composed of the elements Earth and Fire. Its qualities are hot, heavy (but less heavy than Sweet and Salty taste) and it is light and moist by nature. Sour taste promotes digestion, cleanses the tissues, improves absorption of minerals, and it is moisturizing; it can decrease and soothe dryness. It can balance acidity, as well, but too much Sour can be overly heating and can aggravate inflammatory conditions.

Sour taste is grounding for Vata (Ether and Air) especially in winter (Ether and Air) season but can be overheating for Pitta (Fire and Water) especially in summer months (Water and Fire); it is too heavy for Kapha (Water and Earth), especially in the spring (Water and Earth) months. By understanding your constitution and imbalance and keeping the season in mind, you can adjust the different tastes in your meals for a desired effect, and this is precisely how Ayurveda uses food as medicine. Too much Sour taste can be too hot in the summer heat but can provide needed warmth in the winter months.

Sour taste can be incorporated into your meals simply by squeezing some lemon on your food, eating a couple of olives or pickles, or adding a spoon of sauerkraut to your meal. We just need a little bit to awaken our digestion. Some common examples of the Sour taste are sour fruits like lemon and grapefruit. Other foods are sour cream, yogurt, kefir, some cheeses, vinegar, fermented vegetables, soy sauce, and sourdough bread. Fermented vegetables are a viable source of probiotics to heal and to maintain a healthy gut, and to improve digestion.

A small amount of Sour taste adds a refreshing quality to the mind. There is a "wake up" quality to this taste[3] and we can lean into this if we squeeze a little bit of lemon juice and half a teaspoon of raw honey into hot water in the morning. A little Sour taste is needed for us to awaken and too much can feel too overwhelming.

PUNGENT TASTE

The Pungent taste is made up of the elements Fire and Air. Its qualities are hot, dry and light by nature. It is the hottest of all six tastes and most stimulating to the digestion. It creates an increased flow of digestive juices, promoting salivation, and it stimulates the appetite and supports the metabolism. It can decongest the sinuses. It is great for breaking down and metabolizing fats, therefore it is considered catabolic (a process that depletes tissues). Some pungent spices wipe out low grade fungal and bacterial infections as well as intestinal parasites. Due to its cleansing qualities, it is most appropriately added in spring (Water and Earth) time.

Pungent taste is most balancing for Kapha (Water and Earth) as it dries out Kapha's excess dampness and mass. It is least balancing for Vata (Ether and Air), however, small amounts of this taste with other less drying tastes such as Sweet, Salty and Sour is okay for Vata. It can aggravate Pitta (Water and Fire), therefore is better taken in conjunction with other tastes than to avoid it entirely.

Pungent taste is easily added by using the spices for all body types. Fresh ginger root or ginger powder is a great example. A spice mix with just enough kick to stimulate digestion occasionally is fine for all body types.

Pungent taste is found in chili peppers, garlic, ginger, and spices like cumin, black pepper, cloves, basil and asafetida (hing).

Pungent taste is known for its ability to move things. An example will be ginger or cayenne peppers to clear out the sinuses. A little ginger pickle (recipe in Chapter 11) with meals can boost digestion and metabolism.

Pungent taste can bring clarity to the mind and a craving for Pungent taste may point to the need to clear out and let go of past, old issues. Holding past anger, resentment and grudges may become easier if you add some Pungent to your meals. Similarly, reducing this taste may be necessary if one is experiencing a lot of intensity in their emotions.

ASTRINGENT TASTE

The Astringent taste is comprised of Air and Earth. Its qualities are dry, cooling and heavy. The Astringent taste causes a puckering sensation in the mouth. It has a contracting quality and can slow down the digestion. Astringency absorbs water, tightens tissues, dries fat, reduces secretions, controls sweating, settles the stomach and intestines (in some cases), and controls diarrhea.

Astringent taste can cool Pitta (Water and Fire), due to its cooling effect, and reduce Kapha (Water and Earth), due to its drying effect, however. It is not useful for Vata (Ether and Air), as it will make people with this constitution cold and dry. Reducing Astringent taste in the winter months (Ether and Air) is recommended to avoid getting too dry and cold.

There are only a few foods that have predominantly Astringent taste, and these include unripe bananas. Many foods, such as cranberries and pomegranates, have a secondary taste of astringency, as they also have Sour taste. The Astringent taste is secondary in most foods. Some examples of the Astringent taste are herbs like sage, marjoram and turmeric, as well as vegetables like broccoli, cauliflower, artichokes, asparagus, turnip, pears, and dried fruits. Other examples in the grain family are rye, buckwheat and quinoa.

Craving Astringent taste may point to the need to create some boundaries or the need to contain your life and increase focus.

BITTER TASTE

The Bitter taste is composed of the elements Air and Ether. It is light, dry, and cooling by nature. It is the coldest and lightest of tastes. Bitter taste is most medicinal and supports us in many ways. It can reduce inflammation; it's also drying and hardening. It clears damp-heat and detoxifies the liver and gall bladder. It purifies the blood, improves circulation, strengthens the immune and respiratory systems, clears congestion by reducing mucous, supports kidney function and promotes healthy intestinal flora.

Bitter taste is the most underused taste but it is highly recommended for those with Pitta (Water and Fire) and Kapha (Water and Earth) constitutions; those with Vata (Ether and Air) constitution should use it only in moderation, as overuse can be drying and depleting to them.

We don't need to add much Bitter taste to our meals. Just a handful of bitter greens and other vegetables will go a long way. It is a great balancing taste for the heavy, moistening qualities of Sweet, Salty and Sour taste, so adding a little to your meals balances them.

Another interesting effect of the Bitter taste is that it can uplift the spirit by providing a light and flexible energy to our body. So, it lightens the body instead of making it heavy, as in the case with Sweet taste. Bitter taste is found abundantly in leafy greens such as kale, spinach and other vegetables such as Brussels sprouts, broccoli and cabbage. Less common vegetables are bitter melon (see a recipe for this in Chapter 19) and bitter gourd (recipe also found in Chapter 19). These vegetables are most commonly found in specialty grocery stores, such as Indian or Asian grocery stores. Bitter herbs include aloe vera, dandelion, cilantro, coriander, parsley, fenugreek, and turmeric.

A craving for coffee may be an indication you need to add more Bitter to your meals, rather than increasing your coffee intake. And the overconsumption of alcohol may be due to insufficient Bitter taste in the diet.

A craving for Bitter taste generally indicates a need to accept the bitterness or challenges in life and see beyond them. Adding a handful of sautéed bitter greens is a great way to ensure Bitter taste in your meals. It is very useful in summer when we may need some cooling off, and it's advisable to use a little less in winter, especially if you have a small build, are feeling depleted or are underweight. Those with Pitta and Kapha constitution and imbalance benefit greatly from Bitter taste. Those with Vata imbalance should minimize Bitter taste.

To sum it up, Sweet, Sour and Salty tastes are the most balancing for Vata and Pungent, Astringent and Bitter taste are the least balancing. Bitter, Astringent and Sweet taste are the most balancing for Pitta, and Salty, Sour and Pungent taste are the least balancing for this constitution. Pungent, Astringent and Bitter taste are the most balancing tastes for Kapha, and Sweet, Salty and Sour taste are the least balancing. So, reducing what's least balancing and increasing what's most balancing is a way to incorporate these tastes in your meals.

ELEMENTS IN FOOD

Just as different elements make up a different constitution, the same elements can be understood in food as well. When food is treated as medicine, we eat to balance our physiology. For this reason, this part of the chapter is organized by the foods that balance each one of the doshas. Instead of categorizing food as Vata, Pitta or Kapha, they are listed as foods that *balance* Vata, Pitta and Kapha.

One of the balancing principles is to introduce foods with opposing elements. Like increases like. To balance Vata would be to include foods that are opposite to the Vata elements (Ether and Air) which are foods with Kapha qualities. (Water and Earth).

VATA BALANCING FOODS

To balance Vata, we primarily favor foods that are Sweet, Salty and Sour. Since Vata is cold and dry, increasing warm, oily and cooked foods is balancing to Vata. Vata digestion tends to be a little weak and sensitive. It is best to avoid snacking, and instead eat three meals at regular meal times in order to keep the digestion healthy. Snacking gets in the way of efficient digestion, as your body is continuously just burning off what you snacked on, instead of tapping into your body's fat reserves and requiring your digestion to work full-out. Snacking is not a substitute for meals and it's important to only snack between meals if you are really hungry. It is better to eat more at meal times than to snack between meals. Below is a list of the foods in different categories that are balancing for Vata. There is plenty of variety so even if you prefer dairy or gluten-free foods, you should be able to find many options below.

- Beans: Large beans such as garbanzo and kidney beans should be cooked well, with spices and plenty of oil or ghee. All lentils are okay as well and should be cooked with oil or ghee (recipe in Chapter 16) and your choice of spices.

- Dairy: All dairy products pacify Vata. Raw milk (boil before drinking) is the best milk option—if that's not available select organic whipping cream (it is not homogenized and it is pasteurized at a lower temperature in order to be whippable. Add water to the whipping cream and bring it to boil, then cool, before serving.). Avoid hard cheeses. Minimize dairy during spring time, which is a natural time for the body to detox.

- Fruits: Favor sweet, sour, or heavy fruits, such as oranges, bananas, avocados, grapes, cherries, peaches, melons, berries, plums, pineapples, mangos, and papayas. Raisins soaked in water overnight are okay. Soaking will rehydrate them to reduce their drying effect on a Vata body. Reduce consumption of dry or light fruits such as apples (stewed or cooked apples are better), pears, pomegranates, cranberries, and dried fruits.

- Grains: Rice (especially basmati) and wheat are very good. Reduce intake of barley, corn, millet, buckwheat, rye, and oats as they tend to aggravate Vata.

- Nuts: All nuts are good. Soaking them overnight will make them less drying.

- Oils. All oils reduce Vata. Favor more ghee (recipe in Chapter 16), sesame, and olive oil.

- Spices: Cardamom, cumin, ginger, cinnamon, salt, cloves, hing, fenugreek, mustard seed, and small quantities of black pepper are acceptable.

- Sweeteners: All natural sweeteners are good (in moderation) for pacifying Vata. Try cane sugar (also called turbinado sugar), molasses, and honey.

- Vegetables: Beets, cucumbers, carrots, asparagus, winter squashes, zucchini, and sweet potatoes are good. They should be cooked, not raw. The following vegetables are acceptable in moderate quantities if they are cooked, especially with oil or ghee (recipe in Chapter 16) and spices: peas, green leafy vegetables, broccoli, cauliflower, celery, zucchini, and potatoes. It's better to avoid sprouts and cabbage.

Bill came to me as he was constantly feeling bloated; mostly it kicked off in the mornings after he had his steel cut oatmeal for breakfast. My evaluation revealed that his digestion was weak and tended towards constipation (Vata digestion); hence he ate oatmeal in the hopes that it would provide more fiber. On the surface, yes, oatmeal has more fiber than, say, eggs, but in Bill's case, two things were happening. The steel cut oatmeal was hard to for him digest due to his weak digestion and, secondly, the fiber was simply too much (too Vata). It expanded in his body yet did not help move the bowels. I recommended that he eliminate the oatmeal for now, which immediately took the bloating away, and then we started to work on improving his digestion and resolving his issue with constipation. He needed breakfast with more oil or ghee and less fiber, such as stewed apples (Put 1 apple in a quarter cup water, with 3–4 cloves (not garlic), cook covered on medium heat for 7 minutes, and add 1–2 tsp of ghee before serving)

PITTA BALANCING FOODS

To balance Pitta, we primarily favor foods with Sweet, Bitter, and Astringent tastes and reduce those with Salty, Sour, and Pungent tastes. Since an out-of-balance Pitta is hot and can become dry, adding juicy cooling foods with a high water content will balance it out. Avoid hot spices (chili peppers, cayenne, etc.), alcohol, vinegar, fried foods, tomatoes, yogurt, and cheese. Food is best fresh, local, and organic if possible. Avoid leftovers, processed or packaged foods, preservatives, artificial ingredients, and salty foods, as salt increase the two very elements that Pitta is made up of: Water and Fire. Foods with preservatives and leftover foods are hard to digest, making the digestive system work hotter, therefore increasing the heat. Avoid ice in drinks; however lukewarm-to-room temperature beverages are okay. Here is a list of foods that will balance Pitta:

- Dairy: Raw milk (boil before drinking) is the best milk option—if that's not available select organic whipping cream (it is not homogenized and it is pasteurized at a lower temperature in order to be whippable. Add water and bring it to a boil, then cool, before serving), sweet lassi (2 tablespoons of yogurt with 8 ounces of room temperature water, paneer (homemade cheese made from milk (recipe in Chapter 19); butter, and ghee are also good for pacifying Pitta. Reduce yogurt, cheese, sour cream and cultured buttermilk (their sour tastes aggravate Pitta). Minimize dairy during the detox months of Spring.

- Fruits: Favor sweet fruits, such as grapes, cherries, melons, avocados, coconuts, pomegranates, mangos, and sweet, fully-ripened oranges, pineapples, and plums. Reduce sour fruits such as grapefruits, olives, papayas (unless ripe and sweet, as the unripe ones have a tart aftertaste), and unripe pineapples and plums.

- Grains: White Basmati or Jasmine rice, barley, oats, quinoa, kamut, amaranth, couscous.

- Legumes: Mung beans, small kidney beans, non-fermented soy bean products (tofu is OK, avoid tempeh). All other beans are okay in moderation. All beans should be cooked with spices (see recipe for spice mix in Chapter 16).

- Nuts and Seeds: Pumpkin seeds. Blanched almonds in small amounts.

- Oils: Olive, sunflower, and coconut oils, and ghee, are best. Reduce sesame, almond, and corn oil, all of which increase Pitta imbalance.

- Spices: Cilantro, coriander, fennel, and parsley are very good. Cinnamon, fresh basil, cumin, saffron, and cardamom are all right. But the following spices strongly increase Pitta and should be taken only in small amounts: ginger powder, cumin, black pepper, fenugreek (it's bitter and has the secondary effect of a Pungent taste), clove, celery seed, salt, and mustard seed. Chili peppers and cayenne should be avoided.

- Sweeteners: All natural (sugar cane, date sugar) sweeteners are good, except honey and molasses, as they tend to be heating.

- Vegetables: Favor asparagus, cucumbers, potatoes, sweet potatoes, green leafy vegetables, pumpkins, broccoli, cauliflower, celery, okra, lettuce, green beans, yellow squash, and zucchini. Reduce hot peppers, tomatoes, onions, garlic, radishes, and spinach.

Abby came to me due to hot flashes and disrupted sleep patterns. She was in her early sixties and the hot flashes hadn't subsided. She had Pitta constitution and Pitta imbalance. She enjoyed spicy food and happily told me that she thought spicy food was good for her. On top of that, she enjoyed a couple of glasses of wine with dinner. This was a no-brainer; however, giving up alcohol was not something she wanted to do. This is how she and her husband relaxed in the evening and it was more a ritual than anything else. I suggested a substitute drink (made with pomegranate juice and aloe juice in the ratio of 3:1) and had her make a spice mix that was cooling by combining fennel, coriander, cumin, turmeric in the ratio of 1:1/2:1/4:1/4). Along with other dietary guidelines, she started to feel relief from her hot flashes. And, as a bonus, she had fewer nights with sleep disruptions.

KAPHA BALANCING FOODS

To balance Kapha, we need to favor foods with Pungent, Astringent and Bitter taste and reduce Sweet, Sour and Salty taste. Spring herbs and greens such as dandelion greens, mustard greens, swiss chard and kale are good options especially in the Spring. Kapha diet is primarily a warm, cooked, and light diet. Those with Kapha imbalance may not feel so hungry at breakfast or dinner, in which case having only honey-lemon water and a small light dinner is a good idea. Keeping the digestion strong by eating more at lunch time and sipping hot ginger tea throughout the day are good ideas as well. Exercise/movement is a must in order to balance Kapha. Here is the list of foods to choose from.

- Dairy: Raw milk (boil before drinking) is the best milk option. Always boil milk before you drink it, which makes it easier to digest. Adding ¼ portion water and a few slices of ginger to the whole milk before bringing it to boil and adding a pinch of turmeric powder before drinking will make it more digestible and reduces any Kapha-increasing qualities in the milk. Avoiding dairy in Spring time is best.

- Fruits: Lighter fruits, such as apples and pears are better. Reduce heavy or sour fruits, such as oranges, bananas, pineapples, figs, dates, avocados, coconuts and melons, as these fruits increase Kapha.

- Grains: Most grains are fine, especially barley and millet. Do not take too much wheat or rice, as they increase Kapha.

- Legumes: Reduce all beans, especially large beans. Mung beans are okay. As I mentioned earlier, cook all beans with spices (recipe in Chapter 16). A moderate amount of ghee or oil is okay here.

- Nuts: Reduce all nuts.

- Oils: Small amounts of oil only: almond, sunflower, ghee, olive.

- Spices: All are fine, except for salt. It increases Kapha.

- Sweeteners: Honey is excellent for reducing Kapha. Reduce sugar products, as these increase Kapha.

- Vegetables: All are fine, except tomatoes, cucumbers, sweet potatoes, and zucchini. They all increase Kapha.

Carol had gained more than 20 pounds during her menopause years and she had started to feel mental fog, lethargy and depression. This led her to eat more heavy and sweet foods in an effort to feel better, except this caused her to gain more weight and become more sedentary. She had other personal challenges in her life as well, adding to her already stressful life. She did not know where to start. We created a daily routine for her which included just plain hot lemon water in the morning. She never felt hungry in the morning but overate during the day. She would have stewed apple for breakfast, just enough to kick start her metabolism. Adding sweet-tasting vegetables and other items with natural Sweet taste to her lunch —such as dates— took care of most of her cravings for sweets. I recommended a light diet with very little meat and cheese products. With counseling and meditation practice, she was able to get a handle on her stress. Life felt good again and that, in turn, motivated her to keep moving forward. Within four weeks, she had lost eight pounds and is continuously improving her health.

To sum it up, food is also made up of the five elements. To understand which element we want more of and which we want less of is a way to know which foods to reduce and which foods to favor. Just looking at food as good and bad does not tell us much about how the foods add to our health or our illness. That is dependent upon the person who is consuming the food, their predominant tendencies, and their imbalances.

Moreover, the time of the day, the stage of life and the season are all factors that help us adjust the food to the result we want to create. That is why thinking of "miracle foods" and blindly consuming them is a far cry from achieving any real health or balance. Viewing food as such is a naive and fragmented way of creating an effect on our health. Most of the time it leads to haphazard results that don't stick, and don't provide the results that we may have anticipated. Looking at food via its properties, qualities and taste is ancient time-tested wisdom and it has been used to heal and prevent disease for thousands of years. The same still holds true today! When we understand food like this, we can actually use it to create the effect we desire and that is how food becomes our medicine and the kitchen becomes our pharmacy. Open 24/7. What could be better than that?

What is the one taste that you may be overconsuming? Does that happen more in one particular Season? Now relate that to your symptoms. Is there a connection?

CHAPTER 10

Energy, Quality, and Balance

We discussed the foods that balance Vata, Pitta and Kapha in the previous chapter. Now we are going to talk about one of the bigger principles we use in Ayurveda, which is the qualities or energies of the food we consume. This is not the same as the elemental composition of food. Just as emotions affect our digestion, food affects our mood and our emotions. In Ayurveda, we are never just interested in the physical body; rather we take a bigger view and treat the whole person. The three qualities that food conveys are also present in our life and in the Universe. These qualities are Sattva, Rajas and Tamas. When we become conscious, we can choose to either respond (Sattva) or react (Rajas) to our emotions, or we can choose to let go or hold on (Tamas). Let's discuss below the foods that promote these qualities.

SATTVIC FOODS

Sattvic foods help the mind be clear, calm and stay focused. Sattvic food is mostly pure, fresh, organic and vegetarian food, and most of our diet should consist of these foods.

- Alfalfa sprouts, bean sprouts
- All nuts, sesame seeds, sunflower seeds
- Apple, apricot, banana, berries, coconut, cranberries, grapes, honeydew melon, ripe mango, sweet oranges, papaya, peaches, pineapple, plum, pomegranate, prunes, watermelon, and freshly made fruit juices

- Artichoke, arugula, asparagus, broccoli, Brussels sprouts, cabbage, carrots, cauliflower, celery, chard, collards, corn, kale, kohlrabi, lettuce, mustard greens, okra, parsley, peas, parsnips, pumpkin, spinach, summer squash, sweet potatoes, turnips, watercress, winter squash, yams, zucchini
- Barley, beans (black, fava, green, lima, navy and azuki, green mung beans, pinto beans) and green and yellow lentils, mung lentils
- Basmati rice, amaranth, quinoa, buckwheat, millet, wheat, wild rice, oats,
- Butter, buttermilk (fresh), paneer (freshly made cheese), ghee (clarified butter), fresh and pure milk, yogurt
- Fennel, saffron, licorice, cardamom, carob powder
- Raisins, dates, figs
- Sugar cane, raw sugar, maple syrup, honey

RAJASIC FOODS

Rajasic foods generate more fire, aggression, passion and more outwardly-inclined behaviour. Sattvic food can turn into Rajasic food when eaten too cold, too hot and too spicy.

- Avocado, cabbage (raw), chili, eggplant, peppers, tomatoes, radish, red beets, rhubarb,
- Black peppercorn, brewer's yeast, cacao
- Buttermilk (not freshly made), hard cheese and cottage cheese, kefir (not freshly made), olives, sour cream, vinegar, yogurt (not freshly made), pickles
- Chocolate, coffee, green and black tea
- Garbanzo and kidney beans, red lentils
- Grapefruit (sour), lemon, lime, unripe mangoes, pineapple (sour), dried dates
- Malt syrup, molasses, rice bran syrup, jaggery
- Salty nuts and all kinds of salt

TAMASIC FOODS

Tamasic foods are dulling to the mind. They increase inner darkness, confusion and struggles. They promote depression and inertia. Both Sattvic and Rajasic foods can become Tamasic if not eaten fresh.

- Alcohol, all drugs (they act as sedatives, although may be needed for pain) and chemicals
- All meats, eggs, fish, fowl, goat, lamb, lard, pork, rabbit, shellfish, turkey, venison

- Fast foods, fried foods, frozen foods, microwaved foods, processed food, old leftover foods
- Margarine, powdered milk, homogenized milk
- Mushrooms, onions (raw, cooked, green), shallots
- Popcorn, soybeans

To sum it up, food is fuel and the quality of the fuel affects the quality of our life and our mind. This is the reason fresh fruits and vegetables are always recommended for a healthy, balanced life. We can add some Rajasic and Tamasic foods, but only in small quantities. Rajas is the quality of energy, movement and transformation that creates imbalance in life, when in excess, while Tamas is the quality of solidity, heaviness and stagnancy that creates inertia, when in excess. We need all three, however we need them in different quantities. Moving toward a more Sattvic diet and lifestyle will bring the same qualities to your life, bring clarity to your emotions and propel you in the direction of your future. Otherwise, we remain stuck in our emotions and in the past. A lot about a person's diet can be told by how this person is living, thinking and being in the world.

A highly Rajasic person is extremely focused on doing and achieving, and their lifestyle is typical of a modern, "fast" society. Over time, this type of lifestyle causes stress and burnout. A highly Tamasic person, on the other hand, is slow-moving, heavy, lethargic and often depressed. Mental dullness and lack of energy can come about by doing too much, and eventually leads to exhaustion. Therefore, Rajas can lead to Tamas. A Sattvic person is pure in thought, words and actions. They neither overwork themselves, nor are they lazy. We are all part of Nature and we can cultivate the qualities we desire within our tendencies of Vata, Pitta and Kapha. Vata and Pitta can tend towards Rajas while Kaphas can have some Tamasic tendencies. But we can all strive for Sattva because that is what is needed to support our long term health, longevity and vitality.

Hence, the need for balance in all aspects of our life!

Since we are talking about a balanced life and a balanced diet, I think it is important to talk a little more about what it means to be Sattvic. As mentioned previously, Sattva is the quality of Nature that brings about balance, harmony, peace, purity and clarity. And, frankly, we can all cultivate more of these qualities to bring more peace into our lives, homes, communities and our nations.

Food is the biggest factor influencing the energy that predominates within us.

Imbalance or disease is a manifestation of too much Rajas or too much Tamas; too much Tamas can be reduced by adding some Rajas to give it momentum and, similarly, some Tamas can be applied where there is too much hyperactivity, as in the case of Vata. But moving towards Sattva is always a good approach.

Along with food, we can shift a few things in our lifestyle to bring about more Sattva. Yoga and meditation will move you more towards a Sattvic life style. To bring balance is not to change our personality or your preferences, but, rather to put some limits or boundaries on how far towards Rajas or Tamas you will go. Simply having quiet time in Nature can provide an antidote to both Rajas and Tamas. Moving towards spirituality—which is nothing more than starting to connect with your Spirit and your Truth—will go a long way towards creating a Sattvic life. What's important to point out is that we don't want to move towards a Sattvic life in a Rajasic way, i.e. in a "goal-oriented" way; rather it comes about through letting go of any expectations or goals, and simply diving inward whenever possible to connect with your Truth or your Essence.

Another way to promote a Sattvic life style is to avoid crude or uncultured things, such as watching violent and crude movies. Choose uplifting music to listen to; read uplifting things. (Our news programs will not fit into this category). Trust in the bigger picture and expect all good things to come into your life. Watch your speech i.e. the words you use, as words have energy.

What we think about, we bring about. What you think, you digest and it becomes you.

Other things that promote a Sattvic life style are: cultivating uplifting friendships and relationships, avoiding gossip and judgment, finding a work environment that is uplifting, being around like minded people who support your growth and evolution, taking time away from work and other activities that allow you to reflect on your experiences.

Rajas and Tamas present the two extremes of this polarity world. They are an essential part of human life, teaching us to navigate these extremes skillfully and to be in the middle, where Sattva reigns, most of the time. The more we practice, the faster we can move towards the middle. To heal is to have the ability to look at the extremes as they are and maintain a calm and non-reactive mind. A life in the middle is an awakened life. The more we can move towards the middle, the smaller our challenges will be with food and with our life. We are here to heal and as hard as the middle place can be, that is exactly what's needed.

EXPLORING THE MIDDLE PATH

The middle path remains our biggest challenge yet! I think it may be because of this: the middle path asks us to be present and awake, to get over ourselves and see a bigger picture; we are asked to leave the familiar territory of strongly-held beliefs and to enter an unfamiliar terrain of intuition, inner wisdom and trust. Coincidentally, this is exactly what makes our mind/ego feel challenged, become highly active, and vehemently seek to maintain the status quo. In other words, resistance shows up with a vengeance.

Ego/mind was totally silenced when we were swinging from one extreme to the other, even when our deeper self knew something wasn't right. We mistakenly follow the ego's lead instead of realizing that this is the ego's desperate attempt to keep us stuck in old patterns that stopped serving us long time ago. The fear of overindulging in food as a means of comforting ourselves leads us to under-indulge, and food becomes more a nutritional burden than one of life's blessings. When we get sick and tired of counting calories and being disciplined, we swing to the other extreme, tossing all common sense to the wind, only to swing back again, while remaining anxious and fearful. The middle path leads to a balanced state of mind and body or to Sattva.

The fear keeps us in the extremes and the extremes keep us fearful.

The middle path is not about mediocrity, it is a path of heightened awareness and common sense. It is not a path of settling, but rather of choosing the right path for you. Extremes keep us stuck to our limited beliefs and fears. The middle path is one of expansion, wisdom and intelligence. On this path, we know how to navigate the extremes, we know how to detach from our limited mind and beliefs, we know how to expand and look beyond what is immediately in front of us. It is not a path of complacency, rather is it a path of wakefulness.

It is not about giving up, it is rather about finding a higher meaning. It is the path of the spiritual warrior and it invites us to see ourselves in everything and everyone, to rise above our own limitations and connect with that part of ourselves which is infinite and pure Consciousness itself. The middle path is the path of healing, the path of being, of coming into our own human power and potential. This is the path of getting the ego self out of the way and connecting with the real Self. When we move towards the middle, we are starting to wake up.

Ponder this middle path when it comes to food and your lifestyle. What might it look like and feel like for you? Instead of depriving yourself of something you crave, have a little and allow yourself to enjoy it. It is what we do consistently that matters; the same applies to eating junk food. We want to restore our body's innate intelligence in "forgiving" the indulgences once in a while. Enjoy a little ice-cream, or your favorite dessert or snack, without worry and guilt. Similarly, if you enjoy socializing, put a limit on it and make it a special occasion. If spending the evenings on the couch is how you relax after your day, pick a day or two where you find another way to relax, such as going for a walk, doing yoga or dancing to your favorite tunes.

Knowing that we can do these things is a big deal for the psyche; the subconscious does not respond to negatives. When we say, "I can't have ice-cream," the only thing our subconscious hears is "ice-cream." The conscious mind is determined not to have ice-cream, yet we find ourselves eating the last bite from the whole carton. The subconscious mind is subtle but more powerful than the conscious mind, and it hijacks our best intentions. Part of healing our relationship with food is to make conscious what is sub-conscious through meditation, a highly effective endeavor as is mentioned throughout this book.

This is a lot of information to "digest" and it might serve you to consider enlisting a guide to help you determine what body type you have and what kinds of foods will benefit your health the most. To gain a little more insight into your health concerns, I invite you to complete the health questionnaire situated on my website: https://www.ayurvedichealingcenter.com/ayurveda/initial-consulation-questionnaire/.

What is one thing you can do to "soften" the extremes in your life?

CHAPTER 11

Digestibility

Before the use of pesticides, preservatives and genetic modifications, there was not a whole lot of concern about what we ate. We ate what was locally grown and that meant fewer choices. Mother Nature showed us what to eat by what She produced. Processed foods were few and far between. They were enjoyed as treats and no one questioned whether food was good or bad, for the most part. Food allergies and other food-related illnesses were rare.

That's no longer the case. With the abundance of all foods and food products available all the time, many of which are processed, chemicalized and genetically modified, we are sicker than ever. According to the Federal Government, there are 48 million cases of foodborne illness[4] occurring annually in the USA, which means one in every six American becomes sick in this way. Nine out of ten of my clients have a compromised digestion, which results in a high level of toxicity contributing to many illnesses, including depression and other mental disorders.

Our digestive system transforms food into vital energy. More than food, it helps digest our life's experiences so we maintain mental clarity and helps transform those experiences into wisdom. When this system does not work as it should, no transformation is happening at any level, and physical and mental illnesses result. Strong digestion is needed for proper brain function, immunity and mental health. The most prevalent digestive disease is inflammation.

Our digestive system is our body's engine; when the engine does not work, health will fail on all levels. Processed and pesticide-ridden food is one cause of our weakened digestion, the other, bigger, cause is our lifestyle. In the concept of lifestyle, I am including our lack of knowledge and understanding of how our body works, and how to live and eat for its optimum and healthy functioning. This was discussed in the first section of this book where we looked deeply at our disconnect from food, our body's innate intelligence, and our food source.

Processed foods are a big culprit in the development of digestive illnesses. These products are laden with additives and chemicals that were designed to make us addicted to food. "You can't just stop at one," and "made with 50% *real* ingredients" are messages worth noticing. What's more, processed foods encourage a "grab-and-go" lifestyle, and they normalize food addictions and overeating. These products represent not only an assault on our health, but also on our intelligence. How so? They adversely affect our digestive system while suppressing our body's innate intelligence. Advertising companies spend billions of dollars figuring out how to lure us into purchasing these products and they know which buttons they need to push in order to manipulate us into pressing the "spend" button. Instead of allowing ourselves to be blindly maneuvered into buying these unhealthy products, we need to first start questioning whether they deserve to be in our bodies at all. These foods are encouraging us to dumb down. We must smarten up!

The good news is that with Ayurveda's vast knowledge, we can smarten up!

There is so much food available and we have so many food-related choices that it's ironic that we still continue to search for that single food that can fulfill all of our requirements so we don't have to think about it. We look for an energy drink or a food bar that tastes good and is also good for us. It must meet our daily requirements for nutrients and vitamins. It must have fewer calories but keep us full for a long period of time so it can replace a meal. There is too much focus on what we should eat: some of that focus needs to shift to our ability to digest what we eat. Our digestive system, when optimized, can process metal, in the sense that it knows to get rid of what is not good for it. With our lifestyles, we have weakened our digestion to the point where, regardless of eating the perfect foods, we continue to create toxicity in our body.

We are no longer just what we eat but also what we digest and what we don't eliminate. Through digestion we recreate our body. A sluggish, weakened digestion means a sluggish, weakened body!

Food is a causative factor in every single illness on the planet and for that reason it's one of the first areas I address with clients when they come to me with a health issue. This is one of the areas where we can take the reins of our health in our own hands, rather than toss them into the hands of food corporations, and we can shift into that position of strength easily and skillfully.

Food is at the center of life and it is our ultimate health insurance. In fact, food is a metaphor for life: how we do one thing is how we do everything! If we close our eyes to all that food can offer us as a tool for healing, then we are closing our eyes to everything else.

Simple, pure and fresh foods go a long way towards creating better health. We don't need to know or understand everything when it comes to food and nutrition; we can turn the simplest of meals into that which is health-giving. When we can go back to what we already know, pay attention to a few key areas and use a lot of common sense: even the simplest of foods will go a long way towards enhancing our health. In fact, cooking for our health is not about creating the most complicated and exotic meals possible, it is about using our wisdom and our intelligence to create the dishes that will nurture and nourish us.

Peggy came to me due to many health issues, most of them related to chronic pain and inflammation. She did not own a stove and lived primarily on frozen meals. She had a microwave and a refrigerator. She knew that food would be one area where she could make an improvement in her life, but she did not know how. She never bought normal groceries as she did not have the means to cook them, and she really did not know how to cook anything. I suggested that she get a slow cooker and that her shopping list should consist of buying good quality canned soups and beans. I told her that she must walk out of her grocery store with at least two leafy green vegetables of her choice.

I made her a spice mix that she was to use in her cooking. She was able to use the slow cooker to sauté the spice mix, then add canned soup or beans, plus the leafy green vegetables she had bought. She felt like she was cooking fresh food each time she made a meal. She liked her meals so much that she bought a small slow cooker for her work as well. She was no longer eating frozen meals. She increased the variety of the vegetables she used; her menu expanded and she became creative. Using anti-inflammatory spices and foods reduced her pain. She felt more energy and she was very happy with the progress she was making; she also lost some weight.

It really can be this simple. We can begin where we are and move towards health one step at a time. It is never too late to be healthy. We are meant to heal and live our best life. Start today! Figure out what your first step might be, and begin.

Making your own meals for the sake of your health will make you feel engaged in your own life and when we are engaged we are present and enjoy ourselves; this makes us more effective, thus saving time. It is when we disengage that we feel anxious, bored, out of sorts, and unhappy. Start paying attention to this area of your life and it will change your health. The solutions to our illnesses are in our kitchen, not in the doctor's office. And the most reliable way to get the nutrition you need is to prepare your own meals. With so many kitchen gadgets available to help us, cooking is now far easier than it ever used to be. In fact, the act of preparing your own meal is a digestive aid, as the anticipation of eating a meal prepares our body to digest it.

Mental stress and anxiety about food also contribute to a weakened digestive system. What we eat affects our emotions, as we discussed previously. Emotions affect our ability to transform the food we eat into the fuel we need. Stress causes toxicity, even when we consume the most perfect food possible. On the other hand, food eaten with joy and happiness is far more positioned to give us the energy we need, even if it is not the most perfect food. When we are upset or angry, our digestion naturally shuts down to allow us to spend our energy digesting and metabolizing our emotions. It is best to delay eating if you find yourself upset because you might be inclined to overeat in order to suppress unpleasant emotions. This can start a cycle of emotional eating, which is not good for anybody. It's better to just sip some hot tea or sit quietly—your body needs time to digest your emotions. Nothing happens if we skip a meal, and it actually might give your body a much-needed break.

One of the easiest and most potent ways to begin to improve our digestion is to add ginger to our diet. It is a must-have staple in my kitchen and it sits right in my fruit bowl. Ginger is Pungent, and it heats the digestive system. More than a great digestive aid, it settles the stomach and, it's great for colds and flu in the Winter season, it's terrific for allergies in any season and it is a detoxifier in the Spring season. It is highly versatile and it will serve you to make friends with it. Ginger is a medicinal herb that can be used fresh, dried, powdered or as a juice. It has powerful anti-inflammatory and antioxidant effects. It can also reduce muscle pain and soreness. Soaking your feet in water that has been boiled with a few slices of ginger or even adding ginger to your bath, is a great way to get relief from achy feet and an achy body.

Include ginger powder in the spices that you add to your meals. I have added it to the suggested spice mix in this book (the recipe is in Chapter 16). Fresh ginger root can be shredded and sautéed in oil or ghee with your vegetables, and added to soups and stews. Sipping on ginger tea (made with three or four long slices of ginger root and hot water) is a wonderful digestive aid before, during, and after your meals. To add variety to your ginger tea, you can add some fennel seeds (½ teaspoon per cup of water) and/or a pinch of licorice root. Another great way to improve digestion is to eat a couple of slices of ginger pickle before meals. This can be made by just placing some slices of ginger in apple cider vinegar and storing them in a glass jar in the refrigerator. Or you can make fresh ginger pickle by simply slicing a few thin slices of ginger, sprinkling some salt and lemon juice on them, and enjoying them right before meals to stoke your digestive fire.

THE AMAZING GINGER

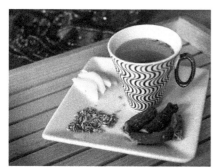

Ginger Tea

Cut up fresh slices of ginger and add hot water. Steep for 5 minutes and enjoy.

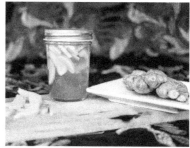

Ginger pickle

Cut thin slices of ginger and add to apple cider vinegar. Refrigerate and have a couple of slices with meals.

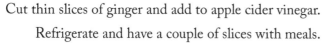

There are many factors that affect our ability to digest. The choice of food, the timing of meals, the food combinations, and the environment where we eat are all contributing factors. Let's discuss them in detail below.

WHAT TO EAT?

- When it comes to food, purity and freshness matter. Choosing fresh, organic, non-GMO food and food in the purest form possible saves our digestive system from being overloaded with foreign substances that it can't recognize. Spending a little extra now to save your future health is the greatest health insurance you can purchase.

- Food left over from a previous meal is okay once in a while but if eaten regularly it can overwhelm your digestive system, as the food is no longer fresh or pure and it accumulates toxins.

- Eat mostly vegetarian and warm, cooked meals. Our bodies do not have the enzymes necessary for breaking down cellulose, which is the major constituent of the outside surfaces of most fruits and vegetables, and cooking makes them digestible. Raw food becomes roughage that lines our intestinal walls, blocking the absorption of vital nutrients.

- Eat the foods that are most suitable for your dosha (constitution), adjusting it according to the seasons and cycles of the day as discussed previously.

WHEN TO EAT

- Eating something light and warm in the morning wakes up our digestive system, warms it up and also helps with the elimination process. Drinking hot water with a bit of lemon and raw honey is a great way to awaken our digestion and get our bowels moving. Morning is the Kapha time and eating something light and warm will balance the Kapha qualities of heavy and cool.

- Eating your biggest meal of the day during lunch time, the Pitta time, is best for harnessing the digestive fire that is available to us during that time and it can provide us with the fuel we need for the rest of the day.

- Eating a lighter meal at dinner time is in alignment with Nature, as it slows down during this time, along with our digestion. In addition, leaving a two-hour gap between our dinner and our bedtime is recommended to ensure adequate digestion while we are still awake.

- Eating at approximately the same time regulates our digestive function and trains our body to work with our natural rhythms and those of Nature. Regularity in meals will make you hungry around the same time and is best for your digestion.

THE ENVIRONMENT MATTERS!

- Eating in a settled environment is good for our digestion. Minimizing the distractions while eating will maximize the enjoyment and satisfaction of the meal. Be present to the different tastes, textures, and aromas, and truly enjoy your food. Allowing that experience to register with all your senses will go a long way towards helping you eat in accordance with your hunger so you do not overeat. Remember, the banquet is in the first bite. A happy and cozy place in our kitchen is an important factor in helping us feel nurtured and nourished.

- Eating on-the-run and while engaged in other things takes away from the enjoyment and satisfaction of a meal and we may turn to other things—or more eating—in order to get that feeling. Your multi-tasking abilities are better served in other areas of your life and not while eating!

- Avoid stimulating conversations, news or phone calls so your energy and attention can go towards eating and digesting. It is okay to indulge in eating in front of a good movie once in a while, but it is what we do consistently that matters.

- A great way to finish a meal, and to have the experience register, is to sit for five minutes after the meal instead of running off to do something else.

WHO IS THE COOK?

Food conveys energy to the body. The food will have the energy of the person who cooked it. So, the level of Consciousness of the cook matters. Food cooked by a corporation—as is the case with frozen, prepared, or fast food meals—is not the same as food cooked by a family member or yourself. The energy of the cook plays a big part in the enjoyment of the food, and it delivers that same energy to us. Have you ever noticed that even when you follow grandma's recipe to a "T," the dish still doesn't taste as good as hers did? Love is a potent ingredient in our meals and that is what's hugely missing in food prepared by corporations.

One of my sisters, who passed away a few years ago, had magic in her hands and in her presence. I enjoyed my meals the most when she was in the kitchen. She knew what I liked, and how I liked it, and she put extra love into the food she prepared for me. One particular time she packed my lunch for a field trip and I could taste the love oozing out of the food she had prepared. A lot of my friends gathered around me for a taste. Luckily, I can say this about all of my sisters especially the oldest one: she not only creates magic in the kitchen but she has the unique gift of making everyone happy with her cooking.

MORE WAYS TO IMPROVE DIGESTION

- Starting the day with stewed apples in the mornings is a great way to kick-start our digestion. (Cut apple into small pieces, with or without the peel, put in a small saucepan and add ½ cup of water and 3-4 whole cloves (not garlic); cover and cook on medium heat for about 7 minutes, checking in between to make sure that more water isn't needed. Discard the cloves, they are added for flavor and to add some heat to the digestion.)

- Sipping hot water throughout the day is a great way to detoxify and help your digestive system stay strong and healthy.

- Eat a couple of pieces of ginger pickle, as discussed earlier.

- Top your food with a teaspoon of ghee (recipe in Chapter 16) and eat it with the first bite to stoke your digestive fire.

- Avoid icy drinks or large amounts of liquid with meals, as the efficiency of our digestive system decreases with cold drinks, and too much fluid tends to liquefy the stomach enzymes and weaken our digestion.

- Cooking with digestive spices (recipe in Chapter 16) helps our body digest and assimilate the food and also helps repair our gut. Digestive spices include ginger, black pepper, cumin, coriander, turmeric and fennel.

- Eating until only 75% full ensures there is some room left in our body for the digestive process to take place.

- Avoid snacking between meals so your body has time to fully digest your meal before it has to digest the snacks. Eating a handful of nuts or a little fruit is okay, however, if necessary.

- Pay attention to how you feel after you eat certain foods. This will help guide you in case there are certain foods that do not agree with you. Notice also the effect of the food on your sleep, mood, and elimination. Our body has its own intelligence and a little awareness can help us tap into it.

What is the one thing you can do to better your digestion? Many times, it is that single step that creates a chain reaction in an upward and positive way.

CHAPTER 12

What Makes Food Ayurvedic?

The purpose of this chapter is to pull all the information together for a practical understanding of Ayurvedic nutrition and also to discuss what may have been left out of the previous chapters. Some Ayurvedic information does not fall into any one category but needs to be discussed. Another key focus of this chapter is to talk about Ama (toxins) in terms of how it is created and how we can clear it up.

What makes food Ayurvedic? Ayurvedic food is not Indian food; however, the terms are commonly used interchangeably because Ayurveda originated in India. This way of cooking and living is common and predominant in India; it's in the culture. But Ayurvedic food is not limited to Indian food. Ayurvedic principles are inherent in Nature and when we respond to Nature in our cooking and eating, it becomes Ayurvedic. Also, food is Ayurvedic if we understand its properties and function and use it to create a specific result. Food is preventive medicine. By paying attention to how we cook and eat, we are preventing future illness. Below are some reminders that may seem obvious, but it is the obvious things that we often miss, and they are pivotal in creating a sustainable change.

FOOD NEEDS TO BE HOT, FRESHLY COOKED, NOURISHING, ORGANIC AND NON-GMO.

A word on why fresh is important: what we eat needs to be available to our body for energy. You may be familiar with the word bio-available, which means our body is able to identify it, therefore making it usable and available for energy. Processed food is laden with additives and preservatives and our body does not recognize them. It therefore does not know what to do with them. Food transforms into energy and waste, and our digestive system must be working well to carry out this process fully. Additives and preservatives cannot be cycled into either energy or waste. Overconsumption of processed food will undermine our body's intelligence and ability to get rid of these chemicals, so they linger in our body adding to the existing accumulation of toxins—or, what Ayurveda calls Ama. The longer Ama remains in the body, the deeper into the tissue layers it travels; ultimately it manifests as disease. Ama is disease waiting to manifest.

Ama blocks the proper functioning of our body; it is like dust on the window which blocks the sunny view outside. Ama blocks our body's innate ability to heal.

The same is true of leftover foods. Cooking for the whole week may be good planning and may save time, but our purpose is to save our health. Although it's better than a drive-thru meal, leftover or old food is not only devoid of Prana (energy), but the food is no longer edible, as it has changed, chemically, from the time it was cooked. Just as with additives, the body can't do much with what it does not recognize as food, and leftovers, in turn, become Ama.

Microwaving food distorts it, so, energetically, it becomes chaotic. Not to mention that leftover foods that have been reheated are devoid of Prana. Consuming these foods also creates Ama.

Genetically modified food is one of the biggest contributors to Ama as our bodies cannot recognize it. What the body does not recognize, it can't metabolize. And what can't be metabolized becomes Ama.

It may appear in our modern culture that most of our eating practices create Ama and hence this is why most people have weakened digestive systems. How do we change that? If we practice living and eating more in line with Nature and our body's intelligence, then we can support what is ideal for our body. We don't get far when we go against Nature, but when we align with it the results extend far beyond what we may have imagined. So, any efforts to create positive changes are worthwhile.

Why must food be hot? Cooking makes food easier to digest. Cooking is also needed to ward off bacterial growth. Hot food stimulates our digestion and wakes it up. Cold food makes our digestion work harder and, over time, makes it sluggish; in that sense it reduces the efficiency of our digestive system.

Cold meals are very common in our culture, especially cold lunches. Those of us working in the corporate world may find the idea of having a hot lunch quite foreign. Chomping on a cold sandwich while working is more the norm. This is where I tell my clients to at least sip some hot water or ginger tea with their sandwich instead of a cold drink. Poor lunches may be one of the reasons people feel extra exhausted from their work day when they get home. Then they eat a long, drawn-out dinner to make up for the lack of proper lunch. Fatigue makes us eat more, and eating while working is fatiguing, rather than as restorative as it should be. A quick way to solve the cold lunch issue is to use a thermos. You can prepare your lunch half way and, while it is still cooking, transfer it to a thermos where it can cook fully and be ready for you at lunch time. Many of my clients do this and love it. Soups and stews turn out great when cooked this way.

SKIP THE COLD DRINKS

Another norm in our culture is drinking large volumes of icy cold liquids during meals. If grease from the dishes clogs our kitchen sink, pouring cold water into the drain will solidify the grease along the pipe and eventually plug our sink. Drinking icy cold liquids does the same thing: it plugs the digestive track—in other words, it creates Ama. On top of that, if we drink a lot of cold water, it will liquefy the stomach enzymes that are needed to break down our food. So, it is a double whammy to have a large icy cold beverage. I recommend my clients sip a cup of hot water or tea and it immediately improves how they feel after meals.

Symptoms of Ama include feeing sluggish, heavy, and lethargic, and having difficulty waking up in the morning. Ama impedes the flow and movement in the body resulting in pain and a host of illnesses. In the same way, our negative emotions, and holding on to past grudges, create emotional Ama that get in the way of our healing and happiness. According to Ayurveda, our declining health has more to do with the accumulation of Ama, and blockages in the transfer of energy, than with age alone. Ama can be eliminated from our bodies through purification methods such as Panchkarma (a five-step Ayurvedic mind and body purification process) and meditation (to purify emotional Ama)

There are a few additional ways to reduce Ama in your body, apart from all that has already been discussed. Here is a simple list of actions you may wish to take:

- Dairy: Low fat milk, lassi made very thin (1 tablespoon yogurt in a cup of room temperature water), ghee (recipe in Chapter 16) and other oils in small amounts, avoiding coconut oil as it tends to be cooling to the digestion.

- Fruits: Grapes, pomegranate, figs, and apples are okay. Avoid sweet fruits such as pineapple, mango, and banana.

- Grains: Barley, rye, millet, semolina, couscous, crackers, rice

- Legumes: Yellow and green mung beans cooked with pungent spices (recipe in Chapter 16) and extra ginger are great. It's also a good idea to make the finished dish a little more watery so it is easy to digest.

- Sweeteners: Honey in small quantities. All spices are good except salt, as it increases water retention and water tends to hold Ama.

- Vegetables: Favor leafy green vegetables and cook them until slightly juicy. Astringent, bitter and pungent vegetables like asparagus, artichokes, radish, celery, zucchini, cabbage, and spinach are good choices. Since your digestion may be weak due to Ama, think about including foods and vegetables that are easy to digest, and leaving out those that are not.

FOOD NEEDS TO BE TASTY AND DIGESTIBLE.

Strong digestion is the key to better health. All of the eating practices and recommendations I'm including here have that goal in mind. We discussed digestion in some detail in the last chapter. As a reminder, it is important to point out that the practices that will stimulate digestion are the ones that turn our food into medicine.

Why must food be tasty? Tasty food stimulates digestion. We begin to salivate just by smelling it and the spices aid greatly in the aroma, taste, texture and digestibility of food. Spices also help bring out the nutritive value of food and help repair and maintain the health of our digestive system.

If we don't like the taste of a food, we are not likely to eat it. Or, if we eat it, we won't enjoy it and it won't benefit us, not to mention that eating something we don't like causes stress. There is so much food available to us that we can all find healthy ways to enjoy food without having to be forced into eating something we don't like. Every now and then, there may be something you may need to do to develop a habit that is going to help you in the long run. Drinking hot water is something some of my clients feel averse to doing, especially if they really enjoy cold beverages, but they feel better with the hot water and this experience reinforces their new habit. More often than not, the results we experience when we make a change in our food-related habits can help us change our likes and dislikes. It also helps my clients when I educate them on the reasons for the changes I suggest.

FOODS NEED TO BE COMBINED SO THE WHOLE MEAL POINTS IN THE SAME DIRECTION.

The example I used earlier of putting grease and cold water in a sink fits here. But, most importantly, we want to avoid combining foods that will hamper our digestion and create Ama. Combining meat and dairy, combining dairy and fruit, combining meals with milk, combining too many ingredients that don't work well together (as in the case of smoothies, discussed in Chapter 3)—all of that will overtax your digestive system and eventually create Ama.

Meat is better combined with green vegetables; yogurt is better consumed without fruits or, even better, taken as a drink with meals (for lassi, mix 2 tablespoons of yogurt with one cup of water). Yogurt is better left out of the meal at dinner time as our digestion slows down in the evenings; milk should always be boiled and drunk away from food, and never with salty meals (it curdles the milk and produces Ama in the body); milk should not be whipped into your eggs to make them fluffy.

As I write this, cheese and meat lover's pizza comes to mind. How about hamburgers, sandwiches made with cold cuts and cheese, and milk with meals? If you are consuming those foods and reading this, don't worry. As horrendous and impossible as it may seem, it is not a big undertaking to take cheese or meat out of your sandwiches or take meat out of your pizza. Start with the idea in your mind and it may not be as difficult as you feel it might be in this moment. Let the idea take seed in your mind. There is a reason why you are still reading about it. Give yourself a chance to shift; your own power may amaze you.

FOOD NEEDS TO BE BALANCING.

Using the principle of balance will go a long way towards stopping us from yo-yoing between diets and fad foods. Balancing meals are created by paying attention to your imbalance, the seasons, the time of day, and eating enough, not too much or too little. It is important to take the time to eat but also not to make it a long, drawn-out affair. Including various tastes and textures will go a long way in satisfying your nutritional needs.

Optimally, 50% of our meal should be comprised of freshly cooked vegetables, including leafy green vegetables. This is easier accomplished if we plan our meals around the vegetables, rather than thinking of vegetables as the side dish. About 25% or 1/4 of the plate, should be whole grains. Many grains are a great source of protein and fiber, they are easy to cook, and very versatile. For non-vegetarians, if you'd rather add animal based protein, then just keeping it to 25% of your meal will reduce the quantity. Adding something sour, e.g. lemon, on your vegetables or soup, or pickles, olives, sauerkraut or a digestive chutney such as mint chutney (recipe in Chapter 19), to a dish is a good way to complete the meal.

FOOD NEEDS TO BE EATEN WHEN YOU FEEL HUNGRY.

Food should be eaten on an empty stomach after the last meal has been digested and not before. Snacking between meals should be minimized and you should only do this if you are really hungry. If you are prone to snacking, it is always better to add a little more to your meals (unless you have blood sugar or other medical issues).

Constant snacking often leads to overconsumption and it gets in the way of fully digesting the previous meal. It is important to mark the end of a meal by washing the dishes and putting them away, cleaning the table, and putting the food away. Leaving food on the kitchen table not only tempts us to snack on it, but it also makes eating a drawn out affair.

FOOD SHOULD BE EATEN IN PLEASANT SURROUNDINGS, WITHOUT DISTRACTIONS OR STIMULATION.

As mentioned earlier in this book, it's important to delay eating if you are upset. This allows complete satisfaction with the meal and curtails overeating.

FOOD NEEDS TO BE BALANCING FOR YOUR PARTICULAR CONSTITUTION.

Food is a big way to change your health. What goes into your body affects your life. An understanding of your constitution and current imbalances provides a deeper understanding of your food choices. This is where it pays to work with an expert instead of risking the errors that may come from using fragmented information or becoming overwhelmed.

Ama results from the poor digestion of food or experiences and it blocks our connection with our body's underlying intelligence in the same way our negative emotions may get in the way of our happiness. When digestion is not working efficiently, food is not properly digested. What is not digested becomes Ama that builds up in our body and our tissues, eventually blocking the channels through which nutrients are delivered.

What is the one thing you can do to move in the direction of eating Ayurvedic meals?

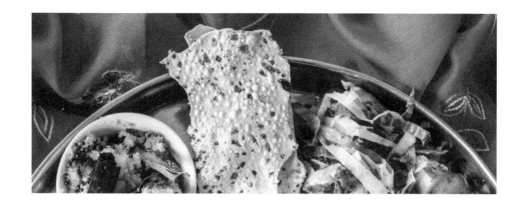

SECTION III

Healing: A Collective Concept

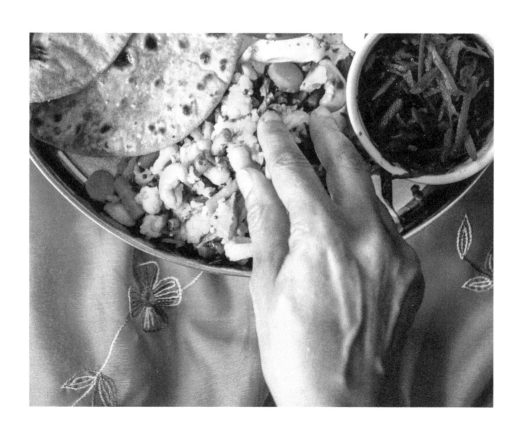

CHAPTER 13

It Takes a Village

Down the street from the house I grew up in lived a family whose little hut was made of mud and straw. My mom knew the family and often talked to the mother when she was out walking. One day my mom came home from her walk and told us that the woman was in labor and needed help. She went into the kitchen to make some special foods for her. I remember my mom making many trips back and forth to this lady's house, delivering food that would help her recover and heal from childbirth. This was very common where I grew up. I remember many other times when my mom would take food to anyone she had heard needed help. There was always a community around us, someone was always coming or going, sharing, and checking up on one another. Neighbors would often share the food they cooked, and we looked out for one another. No appointments were needed; we freely went into each other's homes and kitchens. This type of environment holds the power to heal in a way that no herb or drug can.

I am hopeful that these types of practices are present today in many communities around the world, regardless of how advanced we have become. The need for connection is as basic as the need for air. Love is our true nature and, ultimately, it is love that heals. It is the subtlest yet the most potent force that drives our most desirable behaviour, actions and life, and it needs to be upheld and remembered as if our life depended on it. The truth is, our life and our liveliness does depend on the love in our hearts and in our lives, hence the need to cultivate and foster it in our homes, neighborhoods and communities. Regardless of how much we evolve or prosper, the deep desire for the human heart to connect with another remains.

Many of us struggle with our challenges silently for the fear of shame, or to maintain an image that we have constructed about ourselves. We hesitate to speak up and reach out, especially in the case of mental illness. The truth is that the physical illness only provides a mask for what's going on internally within us. There really isn't a physical illness that is not rooted in our mental and emotional health. We need to be able to converse about our emotional challenges as easily as we talk about our blood pressure or a knee pain. Giving words to what we feel is the first step in getting clear on what's happening internally. Sharing our challenges lessens them; we feel we can breathe again, and find a way to a solution.

We are not our challenges, our illnesses or our struggles. Our human life is the cause of these struggles; they are here to heal us, if we let them. The human life does not differentiate between rich and poor, fat and thin, high or low status. These are man-made concepts or beliefs that have no bearing on our Truth. We must understand that. There isn't anything to hide, as we are all the same in our experiences and challenges.

THE CRY FOR CONNECTION

Our stories may be different but our struggles aren't really that different. If we can understand our own struggles, we can understand the struggles of others. This connection provides support like nothing else can. Even in our spiritual journey, we connect with like-minded individuals who support our growth, understand our challenges and keep us on track. Social media addiction, food addiction, or any other addiction for that matter is a cry for connection. It is a quest for validation and acceptance. "Every man for himself" may be needed sometimes in our lives, but this type of thinking does not really work in the long run if what we are seeking is healing and connection with others. Our desires are not separate from our spirituality; the desires that unravel our human potential are borne of our Spirit. This is our ultimate Truth.

We are alone in our spiritual journey in the sense that we have our own lessons to learn and our own unique path and process to follow, but connection, collaboration and cooperation go a long way towards easing our path and suffering. We don't heal in isolation. We can easily mistake loneliness for independence, isolation for privacy, and create a wall around ourselves. There is a need for deep connection with our heart and its needs; a need to let go of the ego and become real and transparent. We can no longer prohibit real deep conversations and hide behind masks. Our ultimate freedom lies in living our truth. The truth will set you free! Yes, indeed! It is our ultimate shield and defense.

HEALING AS A COLLECTIVE CONCEPT

As we heal, we heal the world around us. Healing is a collective concept; individualism and division does not lead to healing, as our human hearts yearn to connect. We can't limit our thinking to only ourselves, as we are powerful in the way that we affect others, and we are equally affected by others. As we discussed previously, we are part and parcel of the whole of a Creation that includes each of us. Yes, we are responsible for ourselves but we are also responsible to this world that we are a part of. And that is where, as individuals, we can make a shift. What would it be like if the food corporations and the pharmaceutical companies took this to heart and put that kind of thinking behind their products and drugs?

Healing can become an uphill battle when we are dealing with food corporations, school cafeterias, vending machines, fast food restaurants, convenience stores or anything that sells us junk. When the main objective is money and personal gain, regardless of how it is achieved, then global health becomes a challenging goal.

When my son was little, he asked me why cigarettes were sold if they were bad for people. Children have such innocence and wisdom! That is the same question I have. Why would someone sell me something and at the same time tell me it will ruin my health? What if we simply asked that question of the food corporations, who sell us disease-causing products made with questionable ingredients? When people's intentions are to fulfill their personal agendas with a short-term vision, no healing at the global level can really take place. For all the disease-making products and food products that are sold, there is Karma being created and that does not help anyone. I think our world is in dire need of some good Karma. The first owner of the Marlboro Company, Phillip Morris, died of lung cancer. I doubt this was coincidental.

I am fascinated by our obsession with money. How much will be enough? It is this obsession that keeps us all poor in more ways than one, and it keeps us sick, as a nation. Money can be made when you are selling something of value. Why not make money by selling something that promotes health?

The human mind is fickle; it can easily be persuaded or manipulated. It is hard to walk by the racks of colorful, sugary cookies just when you enter a grocery store and even if you do simply walk right on by, there is more persuasion at the checkout line, right in front of you. These subtle suggestions are laid out everywhere in a store, enticing you to bite. This is where our strong connection to our deeply-held desires will come in handy. We can simply smile and walk away. It can't hurt pointing that out to the store managers, if you see them. But as long as we buy these disastrous products, we are helping create a market for them. So, the ultimate responsibility for what's available to us lies with each one of us. If a product is not sold, it does not get made. So, thinking beyond ourselves can fuel our own efforts for healthy eating and living. Instead of being affected or manipulated, we can effect change.

It is not enough to know what challenges there are. It is not enough to be handed solutions, either. One of the obstacles to doing what we know to do is a lack of inspiration and motivation and we need each other for that. Not all of us are self-motivated; some of us need an extra nudge, a reminder, or a little kick, once in a while. Meeting someone at the gym, walking with a partner, and having a pot luck meal are some of the ways that can keep us motivated. Sharing and connecting is how we create a healing community. There is power and inspiration in numbers. However small, we can begin to create our own little village of healing. We must keep moving in an upward direction, as those efforts will be supported by our Higher Self.

"If you want to go quickly, go alone; if you want to go far, go together."

African Proverb

It does take a village. We don't live on an island. We are interdependent and interconnected. We are here for ourselves and for each other. I hope that sharing my thoughts might stir something big inside of you.

How can you create a support system for yourself and perhaps be one for someone else?

CHAPTER 14

I Dream of a Different World

A famous quote from prosperity expert Napoleon Hill says, "What the mind of man can conceive and believe, the mind of man can achieve." The point is that all changes begin with a thought or a dream. In that sense, no dreams are too lofty!

As I come close to finishing this book, I realize it's more than a book. There is a dream stirring in my heart. I dream of a different world; a world that allows healing because it understands that to be the purpose of our human life. Pure Consciousness, the stuff of our making, seeks to express itself in every aspect of our living. And it sees you and me through our pain and suffering. It is beckoning us to grow, to prosper and to shine. Pain is beyond our control, but suffering is something we choose. We can choose Consciousness instead; we can choose to shine like the sun. We can choose to dwell in our own infinite potential regardless of our small-minded agendas and goals. When we can allow Consciousness to simply have us, it will work its magic through us. What if we all understood this? What if we knew that we were more than just our physical body?

Real medicine is that which heals. To divide or to separate medicine into conventional or alternative is to see human beings in a divided, fragmented way. When we do that, it becomes a matter of belief, hence the common resistance to alternative medicine, which gets expressed as "I don't believe in it." I have also come across clients who don't "believe" in prescription medications even when they may need one temporarily.

We can choose to overlook the real root causes of our illnesses, but they remain, whether we believe in them or not. If we believe we are separate from our spirit or our soul, then we do feel separate and fragmented, and are forever missing the deep connection with ourselves, seeking it everywhere, in fact, but in ourselves. When we are fixated on our symptoms, we are viewing ourselves in a rather superficial way, bypassing and missing the opportunities to really become whole. This is what I dream: that we understand who we are, regardless of color, age, sex or creed. Healing happens when we look at the bigger, *whole* picture, it rarely happens when we think we are just a physical body.

STAND UP FOR YOUR HEALTH!

When we become the authority on our own health and healing, we can use the resources available to us in the most efficient and appropriate way. Many times, we must address our physical symptoms to get relief from them, so we can think straight and function, but our focus on health can't end there. When we can step up to what we expect of ourselves, we can use the medical system, both conventional and alternative, in the most informed and effective way. When we stand up for our own health, we won't buy into a predetermined medical system that is laid out before us to blindly follow. We will no longer be lulled into the concepts of health-related comforts and conveniences, but rather rise up to the challenge of facing our fears and becoming whole.

Steve, a 40-year-old man, came to see me. He had had learning disabilities all his life due to an injury during his birth. He managed his daily functions very carefully and methodically. It worked for him.. He lived with his mother but had a job, and he was doing his best. Although he did not completely understand healing, he was drawn to it and that is one of the reasons he came to see me. He also wanted to learn about how to live a healthy lifestyle. Upon meeting with him, I realized that he was actually more functional than he thought. He had a job, he cleaned his home, he did the best he could do every day.

What was getting him down was that he would never be like other 40-year-old men who were married with their own homes and children. In comparison, he felt small and highly inadequate, but otherwise okay with his life. I asked him what it would be like if he lived somewhere where all the 40-year-olds were exactly like him. His eyes lit up and he smiled. By himself and with himself, he was actually quite content. The thought that he was actually okay, or good enough, lit him up. His struggle was not his disability; his struggle was the meaning he gave his disability by comparing himself with others. The revelation that he actually was okay struck him deeply and he looked like a different person. His body perked up, his eyes shone and there was a smile on his face. At the end of his appointment, as he was leaving, he nodded his head and kept repeating to himself, "I am okay! I can do this! This is good!"

Isn't that what we all want? To know, that we are going to be okay regardless of our challenges and our struggles? The struggles don't need to go away for us to be okay, we have to tap into something bigger in us that is far more powerful and potent than our struggles. When we limit a person to their diagnosis, we limit their view of themselves. They become the illness and can't get beyond it. The thinking that we are just our body is limiting and gets in the way of our healing. When we look at illness from the viewpoint of what caused it, rather than how it has shown up, we are creating space to work at its root cause, instead of masking it.

To know that we have created something gives us the power to un-create it.

This motivates us to look deeper, to heal, rather than to give in and succumb to our misfortune. Connecting to our own power is the most healing thing we can do for ourselves.

No one is broken, nobody! None of us are victims! Life is nothing but a series of opportunities for Self-realization. It is up to us to choose to view our challenges as opportunities. How long can we keep running and repeating the same old patterns? Sooner or later, we must step up! I recommend sooner!

The Universe will always support our higher intentions and aspirations, our higher purpose of serving others and spreading goodness in the world. You have the ultimate responsibility for your health. Don't reduce your life to a script and a pill. Your struggles won't lessen with that. Sedating or numbing our minds to the pain will only prolong the suffering. Awakening to our struggles not only lessens them, but will also awaken us to our Truth.

Allow yourself to come alive and to feel deeply, instead or rushing to block your path with a pill. Feeling deeply is your ultimate strength; it is what you can afford to do. Let fear be a catalyst instead of an obstacle. Don't normalize pain and suffering, it isn't why you are here, you are here to heal. There is a yearning in all of us, a fire to awaken to that part of ourselves which is much larger than we can imagine. Connect with that yearning. Nothing creates a bigger burden for our souls than not showing up for ourselves.

Expect more! If you expect to walk away with a script, then that's what you will get. Don't be taken in by dumb and embarrassing marketing. "We call our patients by their first name," the hospital ad says. Seriously? We should drool over that? I like to know what they were calling their patients before. By their disease? The standards have become so low that we actually are impressed if we are called by own first names. The same goes for the standards for early detection, so-called "prevention." If it is detected, it isn't prevented. We must raise the bar as to what prevention is. Prevention is in your kitchen, in how you live. It isn't in a blood test. A blood test is a warning. Why must you need a warning? It is your health, your life, isn't it?

Bigger and filled-to-capacity hospitals are signs of a sick nation and it isn't anything to boast about or to be proud of. I dream of a world where the hospitals become the healing and health education centers. State-of-the art medical equipment, a new wing, and expensive artwork in the lobby isn't my vision. I will applaud when the medical world is concerned more with creating goodwill than collecting patients; where instead of boosting their egos, they are boosting our confidence in creating our own health; where they view the opportunities to make a lasting difference in the lives of those who cross their path, instead of maintaining a limited fixation on their bottom line. The Universe never supports greed or personal narrow-minded agendas; it will always support our big visions and higher purpose. We can, at our individual levels, have a big vision for our health and our life.

I dream of a world where old age is not equated with disease. Disease is not a function of age. We can't have a mindset of being disease-ridden at a certain age. We can't hold on to the cause of death of our parents and their parents. Keep your mind young and keep your beliefs young. Age matters but how you age matters more. Your mindset, and your beliefs, are everything when it comes to your health. Aging is not a disease. If you believe that you are doomed because you are old, then you ARE doomed.

We can run, but we can't hide from our higher calling. When we don't do all that we can do, our soul will seek us out and confront us and we'd better have an answer for it. Live today according to your bigger purpose and calling, and your last day will be a quiet celebration of knowing that you have done all that you could do. You can be the source of guidance and healing. Ultimately, we have to answer to our soul alone, and not to our boss, our CFO or our insurance companies.

I want a world where the healing heart of the physician is more valued than the medical equipment he or she uses. A world where compassion, time, connection and Consciousness are a norm, and not an uphill battle for those desiring to heal. We don't need state-of-the art equipment, we need more healing hearts and hands, a reassurance that we are going to be okay, a reminder that we are more than our symptoms and diagnosis. If the medical world practiced some common sense and wisdom, we might require less testing. The medical processes are more fear-driven than what we truly need. There is more documenting but less listening. Machines can only test what's going on physically, when the true healing is something that happens at a much deeper level. The tests and the x-rays, leave out what's most important: our story, our aspirations, our fears and our challenges, our hopes and our dreams for our life.

The more we accept the system as it is, the more we normalize it. In that sense, we normalize pain and suffering. We have created the medical system that we have today by being complacent and following its development blindly and faithfully. Don't learn how to live with your illness without giving it your all to heal it. You deserve better. It is never too late. We are alive until we take our last breath! Let's not die before our death! We were born to heal, not to suffer.

Imagine the energy and the time we will spare if we are not so vested in our illnesses. We could be immersed in creating something beautiful, learning and contributing to the world. When we connect with our true Essence, we heal. This deep connection nourishes us, and our soul, and we fill up emotionally. Then our life and our eating simply become a reflection of that experience inside.

Can you think beyond your illness? What may your life look like without it?

CHAPTER 15

Food is Our Medicine

Ayurvedic food is distinguished by the fact that it puts a lot of different food items on your plate, offering a variety of tastes, textures, aromas and colors and this is something that is carried over into all aspects of Indian food generally. It truly is a feast for the senses. In fact, it is quite a feat to navigate your way around the meal and it is simply not possible if you are distracted, or even using equipment. The eating experience demands your total presence. What's' more, eating with your hands allows you to taste many different items simultaneously and to feel the food, its texture, and its temperature. It engages your other senses, as well. It compels you to notice the colors and the different tastes and aromas put before you. All of one's senses and energies are turned inward to help digest and absorb the food. This satisfies the inner Self, and eliminates the need to eat continuously. Healing is no different; it asks that we dig in.

On a more scientific side, joining the fingers together to pick up food triggers the most therapeutic and sensitive point in the center of your palm. This releases life force energy to the entire body, enlivening your body and senses for deeper enjoyment and fulfillment.

Another distinguishing factor of Ayurvedic/Indian dining customs is the practice of sitting cross-legged on the floor during a meal. You may have seen at least a picture of that at some point. This isn't due to poverty, although poverty certainly exists in India. There is wisdom behind this tradition: sitting cross-legged on the floor means we put pressure on our stomach each time we lean forward to take another bite. This makes us notice when our stomach is starting to feel full. We start to burp once our stomach is three-quarters full and this signals that we are happily full and at the satisfaction point. Eating anything more would fall into the category of "overeating." Sitting completely upright on a chair acts to suppress this natural sign from our body's innate intelligence.

Growing up in India, I sat on the floor to eat more often than not, and I have carried that habit with me into my adult life simply because I derive more enjoyment from eating while seated on the floor.

Whether you eat with your hands or not, and whether you sit on the floor or at a table, the point is to draw your attention to the immense innate wisdom of your body. Enjoying your food is a must for complete satisfaction and nourishment on all levels. Regardless of how much progress we have made in many areas of our lives, the innate wisdom of our bodies remains, and to undermine, or try to "outsmart" it will only impede our progress in ways that we may not foresee today.

Gaining fulfillment or satisfaction from any area of our life requires our presence. To be fully present to anything, we must slow down. This is an issue that confuses many of us today. We equate slowing down to being idle, wasting time or feeling less important. The fact of the matter is this: time moves at the same rate all the time. How time appears to pass for each individual is a result of their own perception, and it's a direct result of their state of mind. When our mind speeds up, time speeds up. And when our mind slows down, time slows down. When we are mentally rushing, it only feels like we are accomplishing more; it isn't true. We actually are less productive and more frantic and therefore always catching up to the time that seemingly won't stop. So, if you want to slow time, slow your mind. Sit and pay attention to your breath for one minute and notice what happens. Healing on any level is not rushed or scheduled, it has its own timing but it requires that we slow down to notice it when it happens.

Slowing down to enjoy your food will awaken you to the blessing that it is, and that subtle awareness deepens the nourishment and fulfillment it offers. When we can allow food to fulfill these basic needs, we feel full on many levels and we can stop looking to other unhealthy ways to find that fulfillment. When we don't have time to cook and eat, there may be a need to evaluate our priorities.

A few years ago, I visited my sister in Pune, India. Around lunch time one day, I walked outside at the parking level of her building. I noticed many cars and bicycles making their way in to the parking lot, a sure sign that people were coming home for lunch. I could hear the sound of dishes clattering in kitchens and I could smell the aromas of food in the air. There was something very comforting about this: I could feel the energy of slowing down to honour something important: eating.

When we gulp our lunch down in a smoothie, or race through a meal while distractedly paying attention to something else, it may seem like progress, but is it really? I always equate progress to waking up to the innate and ancient wisdom we can all access that will allow us to better our lives and our health. Forsaking our health in the name of progress or success isn't worth much.

Our real hunger is for love, comfort, joy, satisfaction and fulfillment. Food is a medium of expression for all of those vital aspects of what we seek in life. It is up to us to extract the real nutrients from our meals simply by shifting our attitude, by slowing down, and by taking the time that is needed to nurture ourselves. What we experience through eating will be infused into the other areas of our lives. Food is love. Nothing says "I love you" more than a meal that we cook for ourselves or someone else. We feel the love in the comfort, warmth and satisfaction when we eat. When we can allow our ego to shatter and surrender to what simply is, love is all that remains. We heal!

SUPPORTING OUR LIFE ENERGY

No celebration anywhere in the world is complete without food. It heightens every experience and makes it memorable, and we never forget the aromas in our kitchen during holidays and special events. These memories support our life energy. Celebrations in general are about people, connections, sharing and community and the food we serve at these times represents a powerful magnet that brings people together. Sharing is a big part of togetherness—when we like something, we immediately want someone we love to try it. Sharing helps us grow and build connections together. So, if someone asks you to try something, say yes so you can share in their experience.

What if we brought a little celebration into our meals more often? It does not need to be an elaborate effort: celebration requires only our presence. Intention and mindfulness can make every meal more "gourmet" and special. Attention takes as much time as inattention. It takes just as much time to slow down as it does to hurry up. Try it sometime and see what you think.

Anything can heal if used for that purpose and intention. A "miracle food" can turn into poison if used inappropriately or consumed by the wrong person. Many healing medicines in the ancient wisdoms came from the kitchen. There is no replacement for the love and care that goes into that type of medicine and that's a big part of why it heals. Food is our ultimate medicine!

Food is a metaphor for life. How we view food is how we view life. If we view life as a blessing and celebrate being alive and our experiences, food will take us in that direction. If we view life as a curse or difficult, no amount of food will sweeten our experiences of life. Food is not separate from life and life is not separate from food. If we believe we are here to heal, we will naturally consume the food that will heal us.

Food has been used to correct imbalances, treat illnesses, and reverse aging and it is at the core of vitality and longevity. It connects us to the very essence of life, and using its wisdom is the key to our health and happiness.

We are living in blessed times indeed where our kitchen appliances and gadgets make much of our food preparation work easy. What's more, food is available all the time. There has never been a time when the ancient healing wisdom of food can serve us so powerfully and in ways that are far beyond our imagination.

"Let food be thy medicine and medicine be thy food"

Hippocrates

Food is the most natural state of medicine, providing healing energy with every bite. It repairs our internal organs, nourishes our body, and comforts our soul. Our body's own innate intelligence guides us as to what to eat if we don't get in the way. It is more common-sensical than we think. Paying attention to the effects of food on your mind, body and soul can create a solid frame of reference that will point the way to which foods are good for you and which are not. Food is a tasty way of restoring balance to your body. Believe in the healing power of food and you will naturally be drawn to use food in this way.

The most reliable source of strength in challenging times is our health, and self-care is an important part of this. Think about cooking and eating as part of your self-care. Check your grocery cart, your pantry, your refrigerator and your dinner plate.

Does the food you have in your grocery cart, in your kitchen, or on your plate fulfill the promise of health and healing?

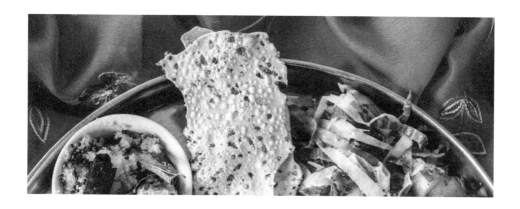

SECTION IV

Recipes:
Let the Healing Begin
in Your Kitchen

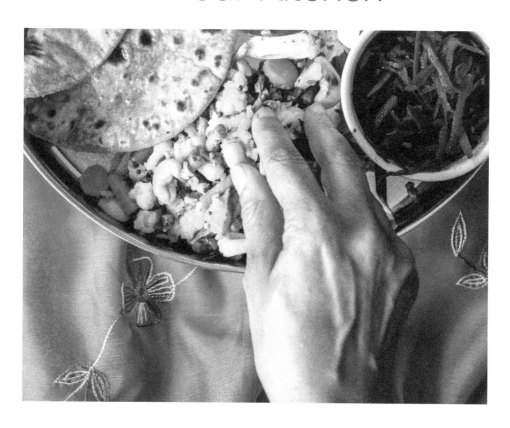

CHAPTER 16

Stocking Your Ayurvedic Pantry

little planning goes a long way in creating mindful and healthy meals and having the ingredients you need available right in your pantry can make meal preparation easy and joyful. You may have your own way of stocking your pantry and your own shopping rhythm and ritual. I normally buy fresh vegetables and fruits perhaps twice a week and I stock many other items well in advance, as they can keep longer. Here is a list that I have categorized under different headings to help me remember what I have and what I need. You don't need to have all the items all at once, you can start with few items and can build from that.

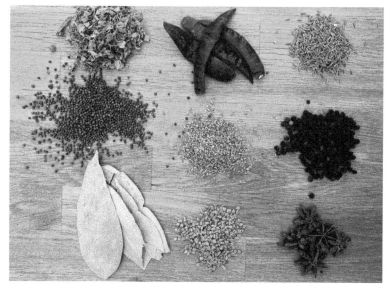

SPICES

Not only do spices make food more interesting and enjoyable but they turn food into medicine and bring the healing intelligence of food to our table. Spices awaken our senses and add many dimensions to our meals. You will want to have on hand the following:

Asafetida, black pepper (whole and ground), cumin seeds, cardamom powder, cinnamon powder and sticks, bay leaves, cloves, coconut (flakes and pieces), coriander seeds, cumin seeds, fennel, fenugreek (seeds and dry leaves), ginger powder, mineral salt, mustard seeds, pomegranate seeds, saffron threads, tamarind, turbinado sugar, turmeric powder, whole green and black cardamom.

OILS AND GHEE

Coconut oil and safflower oil for high heat, olive oil for low heat; ghee (clarified butter) can be used for both low and high heat; use avocado oil for high heat and it's also great for salad dressing. You'll find the recipe for ghee below.

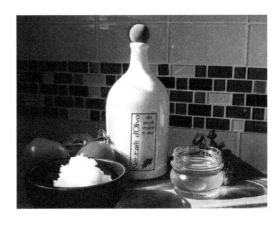

GRAINS

Amaranth, barley, basmati Rice, brown rice, buckwheat, oats, pasta, quinoa, tapioca

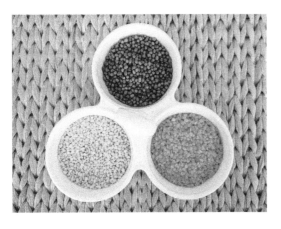

LENTILS/LEGUMES

Brown, green, orange and yellow lentils

Black-eyed peas, black beans, black chick peas, garbanzo beans, kidney beans, split peas

FLOURS

All-purpose flour, almond flour, chapati flour, chick pea flour (besan), semolina (sooji)

NUTS/SEEDS

Almonds, Brazilian nuts, cashews, pine nuts, pistachios, walnuts

Chia seeds, flax seeds, hemp hearts, sesame seeds, sunflower seeds

FRESH FRUITS AND VEGETABLES

Buying fresh vegetables and fruits once or twice a week is best. Always have ginger, lemons and leafy greens, and a few fresh pieces of fruit, to enjoy throughout the week. Buy foods with vibrant colors.

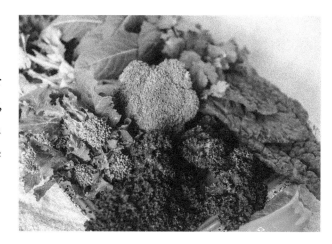

GHEE AND SPICE MIX

These two items can be made beforehand so you always have them available. Here are recipes for both:

GHEE

Ghee is clarified butter and it is most nourishing to the nervous system. Enjoy a little teaspoon with the first bite of any meal to stoke your digestive fire.

1. Place 4 sticks of butter (16 ounces or 2 cups) of unsalted organic butter in a medium pot on less-than-medium heat, uncovered.
2. Once the butter melts, the water contained in the butter will start to boil and make a distinctive sound.
3. Continue boiling for about 12-15 minutes. The milk solids will settle to the bottom of the pot, and the ghee will start to crackle with a high-pitched sound.
4. Turn the heat to low and continue cooking for another 5 minutes. You will see the golden yellow liquid in the middle and foam around the sides of the pot.
5. Don't overcook, as the liquid can easily burn and turn dark.
6. Turn the heat off and let cool for 10 minutes.
7. With a spoon, skim the foam crust off or push it to the side and pour ghee into a glass jar. Or you may use cheesecloth to strain the ghee into a glass jar.
8. Ghee does not need to be refrigerated. It will keep fresh on the countertop. Use as needed.

SPICE MIX

Make a small batch as fresh spices are more potent.

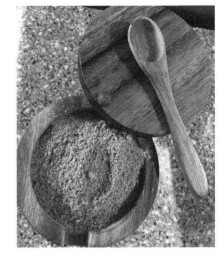

1. Grind half a cup of fennel seeds, ¼ cup cumin seeds, and ¼ cup coriander seeds together in a spice grinder.

2. Pour the mixture into a bowl.

3. Add ⅛ cup turmeric powder, 1 teaspoon ginger powder, ½ teaspoon black pepper powder, ½ teaspoon of asafetida (hing), and dash of salt. .

4. Mix ingredients together and store in a glass jar in your cupboard.

5. Always start with a small amount to test; you can always add more to the dish you are preparing.

CHAI SPICES

Cinnamon, cloves, cardamon, black cardamon, fennel, fresh ginger root
Recipe on page 189.

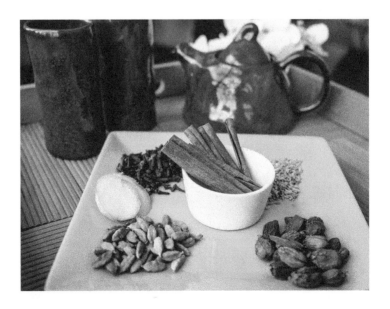

CHAPTER 17

Be Your Own Master Chef

When hunger strikes, we are all sufficiently equipped to figure out a way to eat. That need serves as the basis for all of us to become creative in the kitchen and make our own recipes based on what we have and what we feel like eating. Now, with your new-found knowledge of food as presented in this book, and a mindfully-stocked pantry, you can create healthy dishes in no time. Navigating your own kitchen and taking care of your basic need for food, energy and nourishment is a great skill and will give you a feeling of accomplishment and joy. Self-reliance is a much bigger confidence booster than chasing another recipe or a food fad.

We can always get our meal from a box, the freezer, or a fast-food restaurant, but something greater than just the nourishment is amiss when we do that. The quality of our life is the sum total of our experiences. Short cuts are needed sometimes, but the richness of life comes from taking the longer route. This is a journey we can take right there in our own kitchen. As I mentioned before, chopping, stirring and tasting will not only give you the nourishment you need, but it will also add joy and satisfaction to every meal you consume. Immerse yourself in the experience and see what happens.

The process of meal preparation, setting up the table and creating a calming and inviting environment nourishes us on more levels than just the physical. Here are a few things to keep in mind as you forge forward in your kitchen. The more we are at ease in the kitchen and preparing healthy foods, the less reliance we place on the food corporations to do that for us.

1. Keep food simple. Simplicity attracts wisdom! One of the things I learned from my father is that **simple living leads to high thinking**.

2. Simple dishes are richer in taste and nourishment. Our physiology recognizes and understands

the simple tastes and ingredients better than the complex ones, and it works seamlessly to extract nutrients from it. Simplicity and goodness go together like a slice of fresh bread and butter with your favorite herb or spice sprinkled onto it. When it comes to food, less is always more: the fewer ingredients you use the better tasting the food is.

3. Recipes provide the basic foundation for a dish and many require special ingredients to make them just right. However, they can be daunting if we don't recognize the ingredients or we don't have them on hand. Always practice one new recipe at a time. Get a general idea about what you are cooking from the recipe itself but be willing to be creative about it. Add something new, take something away. Allow your senses, and your intuition, to guide you, and just flow with it. Be willing to mess around and create. If the dish does not turn out well, and you don't like it, there is always pizza! **There is no perfection, only a process.**

4. Cooking is mostly an art with a little bit of science. By understanding the basic science of cooking, and combining flavors, there is a lot of room to play and create. Experienced cooks don't measure, or follow specific steps, they create mostly by feel. Cultivate that in your cooking by being playful, veering away from the recipe and allowing your own creativity to kick in. Improvise, substitute, and add more or less of an ingredient. You never know what you might invent. Allow your senses to guide you. The worst-tasting dish will teach you the most. Experimenting is what makes cooking fun and joyful.

5. Is this good for me? Is this okay to eat? Let your experience guide you. All of us are equipped to know how eating something makes us feel. We don't need any scientific research to validate our experience. Trust your own experience. Tune into your body. What do you feel like eating? What taste? What texture? Go for it! Don't force yourself to eat something just because you believe it is good for you. The enjoyment of food is an important ingredient in your healing journey. With the abundance and variety of foods available today, we can all find many different foods that we like and enjoy.

6. Let your kitchen be a place of joyful memories, rich aromas, laughter and healing. Go out for the evening, in your kitchen.

7. There are many things we have to be serious about in our lives, but cooking does not have to be one of them. Approach it lightly and playfully. Food is our medicine and the kitchen is our pharmacy! Engage your senses, taste as you eat, play your favorite music, light a candle, add a bit of this and that, chop, grind and mix. Make your own recipe from what you have in the fridge and the pantry. How do you think I came up with the recipes here? There is planning, then there is play. Leave room for play!

8. Don't forget the most important part! To sit down, enjoy your creation and relax! Don't contain your enjoyment, express it freely! This positive experience will reinforce your efforts and invite you to continue to play in the kitchen.

CHAPTER 18

Notes About the Recipes

1. This book contains only a handful of my favorite and frequently-made recipes, enough to get you started on healthy Ayurvedic meals. They are presented in alphabetical order, using the translated English names (which mostly are the names of the main ingredients). The Indian names are included in parenthesis where possible.

2. The recipes are balancing for all doshas unless otherwise specified in the comments section of each recipe.

3. Most recipes can be enjoyed for either lunch or dinner, with a few exceptions. To make it easy for you, I've categorized the recipes as suitable for B (Breakfast), L (Lunch), D (Dinner), C (Chutney or Sauce), HB (Hot Beverages), and S (Sweets/Dessert). You can also refer to the index to find recipes under each section.

4. I have organized the ingredients in table form so you will have an "at-a-glance" idea of all that you may need to collect before trying the recipe. Some of the "ingredients" such as a pot or a pan may be obvious to some of us who are very comfortable in the kitchen, but I am hopeful the novices among us will become comfortable and self-reliant in the kitchen as well, so I have listed those items under the "Kitchen Gear" column. I've excluded the more common gear such as a knife or a cutting board, but please note they are needed for almost every recipe.

5. You don't need a lot of complicated kitchen gear. Here are the items that you are most likely to need:
    *   2 -3 medium saucepans with lids
    *   a small frying pan to prepare tarka
    *   2 medium pots

- a kadai (this is a thick rounded pan used mostly in Indian cooking for deep frying)
- a tawa (this is another Indian flat disc-shaped frying pan to make chapati, Indian flat bread; you can improvise by just using a non-stick frying pan)
- 1-2 mixing bowls, a cutting board, a sharp knife, large serving spoons, a rolling pin, a blender, a small food processor, small containers for storing spices.

6. The "Herbs and Spices" column you'll find with each recipe includes things like sugar, salt, baking powder etc., unless that is the main ingredient in a recipe. My cookie recipe is the only one where sugar is one of the main ingredients and therefore sugar moves to the "Main Ingredients" column for that one. I've included in the "Herbs and Spices" column anything that adds accent, flavor, or texture to the main ingredients, such as salt. It is not an herb or a spice, but is included in the herbs and spices column as it can't be in the main ingredient column. You may notice some inconsistencies in the recipes depending on how the items are used.

7. Cooking is not an exact science. If it were, it would take all the fun and creativity out of it. I learned to know the right amount of an ingredient instinctively by the smell, color and texture of the dish, and by experimenting. I seldom measure any ingredients and it was humbling to work backwards for this book to find exact measurements. Regardless, there is room to play in the recipes and to be creative. You will notice that I have provided a range of amounts for some ingredients and I invite you to adjust to your preferences. If cooking with spices is new to you, then I recommend using the lower range to start; you can always add more according to taste. The same is true of ghee or oil. If you like your dishes to be a little more oily (and some dishes taste better, and are more nourishing, when more oily, as I've mentioned in some recipes where that applies) adjust accordingly. Preparation times and serving sizes are also approximations.

8. I refer to two techniques in some of the dishes.

- **The first one is Tarka.** Tarka is a way to maximize the flavor of spices before adding them to the food, and to infuse flavor, aroma, richness and color into the dish. Tarka is prepared in a small pan separately from the main dish, in the case of liquid dishes and soups. In the case of dry vegetable dishes, Tarka is prepared in the pan to which the vegetables will be added. Tarka is prepared by always heating oil or ghee in the pan for a few seconds before adding the spices. I prefer medium heat so the oil or ghee does not burn. If the dish calls for onions, tomatoes or ginger, the onions are cooked first to extract their flavor. Tomatoes and ginger are added next and cooked for the specified time. In order for the medicinal qualities of the spices to come though, it is important to cook them in oil or ghee. To make sure there is enough ghee or oil for the spices to cook, we generally push the mixture (of onions, tomatoes, or ginger, as the case may be) to one side to drain the ghee to the center; then we add spices to that ghee. When the spices splutter or bubble, they are done and we can mix them with the rest of the ingredients in the pan (often tomato, onion, and ginger) before adding to the main dish, or before adding the vegetables, depending on the recipe. This is often accompanied by a sizzling sound that signifies the distribution and infusion of flavor into the dish. The resulting aromas prepare your body to receive the food and digest it well.

- **The second technique is Condensation.** This I learned from my sister in Pune, India. This technique is used for dry vegetable dishes. The pan is covered with the lid turned upside down. We add a little bit of water to the lid and the steam and heat from the pan creates condensation, allowing the water to be added to the dish a few drops at a time as needed, so the vegetables don't burn and they are not watery. A couple of teaspoons of water is sufficient.

9. Ghee is revered in Ayurveda due to its neurological and digestive qualities i.e. it is highly beneficial for our nervous system and a little bit eaten with the first bite can stoke our digestive fire. Ghee is cooling and calming. It is great to add a bit more in Winter months when our bodies tend to be dry; a little bit in the Summer months can be cooling. It is best to minimize ghee and use only what's needed for cooking in the Spring. You will notice a range given in the recipes that you can adjust according to your taste and the season. A little ghee added to a dish makes it very tasty, so don't be afraid to add more.

10. The steps in most of the recipes are the same. We always start with oil/ghee in the pan, add the base for Tarka, onions, tomatoes and whatever else is suggested, then add the spices so they splutter a little, which only takes 15-20 seconds. Be careful that you don't burn the spices, but if you do, you can start over. If the ingredients aren't ready, you can always turn the heat off, or remove the pan from the heat until the other ingredients are ready.

11. Unless otherwise specified, I suggest cooking on medium heat and turning the burner down a little once all the ingredients have been added. High heat tends to dry and burn dishes without cooking them. It is okay to start with high heat so the dish can get sufficient heat for cooking and then turn the heat down to medium.

12. Most dishes are served with rice, chapati or a bread of your choice. Feel free to eat them alone, and mix and match as you like.

13. Most recipes have pictures which I hope will inspire you to enjoy the process of cooking even more!

CHAPTER 19

Recipes

 BREAKFAST

- Energy Balls
- Fruit and Nut Bowl
- Savory Chick Pea Pancake
  (Besan ka Purah)

 LUNCH

- Chick Pea Flour and Yogurt Dish
  (Karhi Pakora)
- Hearty Spiced Chick Peas (Kabuli Cholley)
- Vegetable Fritters (Pakorah)

 LUNCH AND DINNER

- Bitter Gourd with Kale (Gheeya)
- Bitter Melon (Karela)
- Black Chick Peas (Kala Chana)
- Cabbage with Potatoes and Peas
  (Band Ghobi Aloo)
- Cranberry, Black Pepper, Cashew Rice
- Cumin Basmati Rice (Jeera Chawal)
- Eggplant with Peas (Bharta)
- Ginger Soup (Adarak ki Tari)
- Green Lentil Soup with Celery
  (Sabut Mungi ki Daal)
- Homemade Cheese and Pea Curry
  (Mutter Paneer)
- Indian Flat Bread (Chapati)
- Lentil and Rice Soup (Khicharhi)

- Okra (Bhindi)
- Rapini and Broccoli Saag (Sarsaun Ka Saag)
- Rice with Vegetables and Nuts
- Spiced Mixed Vegetables (Sabji)
- Spinach with Lentils (Daal Paalak)
- Spring Black Eyed Pea Salad
- Stove Top Acorn Squash (Kaddu)
- Turmeric Pasta with Pan-Grilled Vegetables
- Turnips and Spinach (Paalak Shalgum)
- Yellow Lentils (Moongi ki Daal)

 SWEETS

- Chick Pea Burfi
- Energy Balls
- Four C's Pudding
- Smart Cookies
- Tapioca, Chia, Hemp Seed Pudding

 CHUTNEYS

- Coconut Chutney (Nariyal Chutney)
- Mint Chutney (Pudeene Ki Chutney)
- Raisin Date Chutney
- Tamarind Sweet and Sour Chutney
  (Imlee Ki Chutney)

 HOT BEVERAGES

- Almond Date Shake
- Spiced Tea (Masala Chai)
- Golden Milk (Haldi ka Dhoodh)

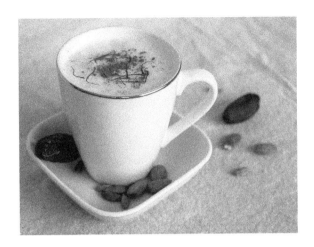

ALMOND DATE SHAKE

A nourishing treat! Great for winter mornings or winter nights. Soothing and comforting!

• Preparation time: 10 minutes

• Serves 2

Main Ingredients	Herbs/Spices	Oil/Ghee	Kitchen Gear
2 dates	A sprinkle of cardamom powder		2 Small bowls
10 almonds	A few strands of saffron		Medium pot
2 cups of milk*			Blender

*can substitute with milk of your choice

Directions

1. Soak dates and almonds in separate bowls overnight in water (soaking makes them easier to blend).

2. Peel the almonds (and dates, if necessary: they may have a thick peel that you can remove), and remove the pits from the dates.

3. Boil milk.

4. Add the almonds and dates to blender with half the milk. Blend until the ingredients are puréed. (Adding only half the milk ensures that the almonds and dates puréed well.)

5. Add the rest of the milk to the blender and give it another quick buzz.

6. Pour into cups, then garnish with cardamom powder and saffron threads.

Enjoy!

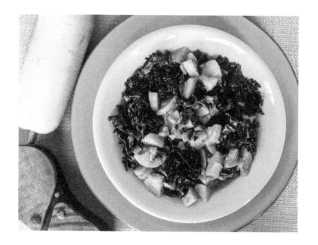

BITTER GOURD WITH KALE (GHEEYA)

A light and slightly bitter dish, great for spring and summer meals.

• Preparation time: 20 minutes

• Serves 4

Main Ingredients	Herbs/Spices	Oil/Ghee	Kitchen Gear
1 bitter gourd or zucchini	½-1 teaspoon salt	2-3 tablespoons of ghee*	Medium pan
2 cups water	1 teaspoon spice mix*	or coconut oil	with lid
4 stalks of kale			
1 teaspoon shredded ginger			

*recipe in Chapter 16

Directions

1. Peel the bitter gourd, cut it in half lengthwise, remove the soft middle, and then cut it in small pieces. If you are using zucchini, chop in half rounds that are about an inch thick.

2. Put ghee in the pan and heat on medium for 15 seconds. Add ginger and spices and cook for another 15 seconds.

3. Put gourd or zucchini in the pan, mix it with the spices and add 2 cups of water.

4. Cover the pot and cook on medium heat for 10 minutes.

5. The gourd is cooked when it darkens in color. If you are using zucchini, you may need to cook it for less time, about 7 minutes.

6. Rinse kale thoroughly with fresh water. Strip it kale from the stems and break the leaves into small pieces.

7. Add kale to the pan, then cover and cook for another 2 minutes.

8. Mix well and serve hot.

Enjoy!

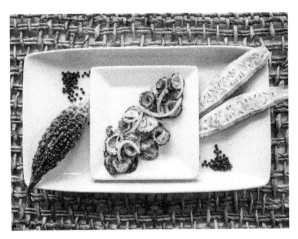

BITTER MELON (KARELA)

This vegetable has a special place in Ayurvedic medicine. With its bitter taste, it is light and quite beneficial for inflammation and diabetes. Serve with lentil soup in small portions. Great for spring and summer meals.

• Preparation time: 20 minutes

• Serves 2-4

Main Ingredients	Herbs/Spices	Oil/Ghee	Kitchen Gear
2 bitter melons (karelas) 1 small onion, cut in long and thin slices	¼ teaspoon turmeric ¼ teaspoon salt ½ teaspoon mango powder	2-3 tablespoons coconut oil	Paper towel Small frying pan Bowl

Directions

1. Coarsely scrape away the prickly parts of the karelas with a regular knife and wash.

2. Dry with a paper towel.

3. Cut the karelas in half lengthwise and scoop out the seeds if they are red or too hard. If they are soft, you can leave them.

4. Cut the karelas in small, thin slices.

5. In a frying pan, heat coconut oil on medium heat and fry slices of kerala until lightly brown.

6. Pour contents of the pan into a bowl.

7. In the same pan, sauté onion until light brown. Add turmeric, mix it with onions.

8. Now add fried kerala pieces to the pan. Mix well. Add salt and mango powder. (Adding sour mango powder reduces the bitterness of the karelas.)

Enjoy!

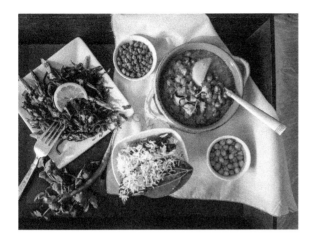

BLACK CHICK PEAS (KALEY CHOLLEY)

A hearty, nourishing and satisfying dish, this is a great source of protein and fiber. Enjoy with rice or chapati. Since chick peas tends to be drying, it is better to add a bit more ghee to this dish. This is a great dish to consider when you are feeling run down or depleted.

- Preparation time: 20 minutes (plus time for soaking and boiling)
- Serves 4-6

Main Ingredients	Herbs/Spices	Oil/Ghee	Kitchen Gear
2 cups dried black chickpeas	3-4 bay leaves	5-6 tablespoons of ghee*	Slow cooker
10-12 cups water	1 teaspoon cumin seeds		Food processor
1 chopped tomato	1 teaspoon coriander seeds		Serving spoon
1 small onion, minced	1-2 teaspoons spice mix*		Small pan
1 teaspoon grated ginger	1 teaspoon turmeric powder		
¼ cup chopped cilantro	⅛ hing (asafetida)		
1½ chopped green chili peppers (optional)	1½ teaspoons salt		

*recipe in Chapter 16

Directions

1. Soak dried chickpeas for a minimum of 4 hours in warm water. Rinse with fresh water and place in slow cooker with 10-12 cups fresh water. Add bay leaves. Set the slow cooker to high heat for 4 hours. Cook until soft. Add a little more water if dry.

2. Mash some of the chick peas on the sides of the cooker with a serving spoon. This will make the gravy a little thicker.

3. Heat ghee in small pan for 15 seconds; add minced onions and sauté until brown. After the onions are brown, add tomatoes and grated ginger. Cook for 3-5 minutes on medium heat.

4. Push the mixture to the side of the pan and allow the ghee to pool in the bottom. Add cumin and coriander seeds, let them splutter, and then add the spice mix, turmeric powder, and salt. Cook for another 15 seconds. Mix and cook for another 2-3 minutes.

5. Add this mixture to the slow cooker. Mix it well and serve it hot. Garnish with cilantro and a dab of ghee.

Enjoy!

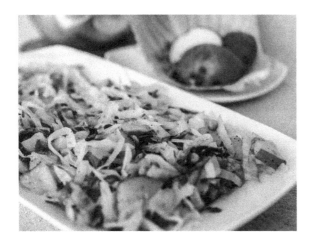

CABBAGE WITH POTATOES AND PEAS (BUND GHOBI ALOO)

This is a light and slightly bitter side dish, usually served with chapati or rice. Adding potatoes and peas balances out the bitter cabbage.

- Preparation time: 15-20 minutes
- Serves 2-4

Main Ingredients	Herbs/Spices	Oil/Ghee	Kitchen Gear
½ small cabbage	1 teaspoon shredded ginger	2 teaspoons ghee*	Flat pan with lid
1 potato	1 teaspoon cumin seeds		
1 teaspoon water	½ teaspoon turmeric powder		
½ cup frozen peas			

*recipe in Chapter 16

Directions

1. Cut cabbage into long thin strands and dice potatoes into medium pieces.
2. Put ghee in the pan and let it heat on medium for 15 seconds. Add ginger and
3. cumin. Cook for 15 seconds.
4. Add potatoes and a teaspoon of water. Cover the pan and cook for 5 minutes on
5. medium heat.
6. Add cabbage and stir. Cover the pan and cook for another 5 minutes.
7. Add peas and mix. Cook for another 2 minutes.

Enjoy!

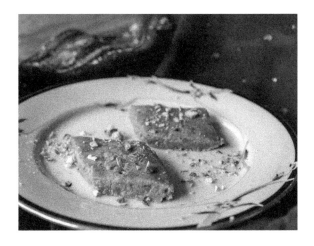

CHICK PEA BURFI (BESAN BURFI)

Think of this as a modern day protein bar. It has the purest of ingredients, and it's great as a snack with tea, as a desert, or as a quick breakfast.

- Preparation time: 15 minutes
- Makes 10-12 pieces, can be stored in the pantry

Main Ingredients	Herbs/Spices	Oil/Ghee	Kitchen Gear
1 cup besan (chick pea flour) Slightly less than ¼ cup sugar	2 teaspoons chopped pistachio nuts 2 tablespoons milk	½ cup ghee*	Heavy-bottomed pan Flat metal plate

*recipe in Chapter 16

Directions:

1. Heat pan on medium.
2. Add ghee and besan to the pan, and stir.
3. Once the ghee has melted, turn heat to low.
4. Stir slowly and continuously for about 10 minutes.
5. When you begin to smell the mixture, you know that it is cooked. Another sign that the mixture is cooked is that the ghee will begin to separate from the mixture. Test by adding a touch of extra ghee. If it separates instead of soaking in, cooking is complete.
6. Turn the heat off, add sugar, and mix.
7. Add milk and mix.
8. Pour the mixture into a large pie plate (Be careful if using a non-metal plate as the heat can break the plate).
9. Let mixture cool for at least 20 minutes.
10. Garnish with pistachios.
11. Cut in diagonal pieces.

Enjoy!

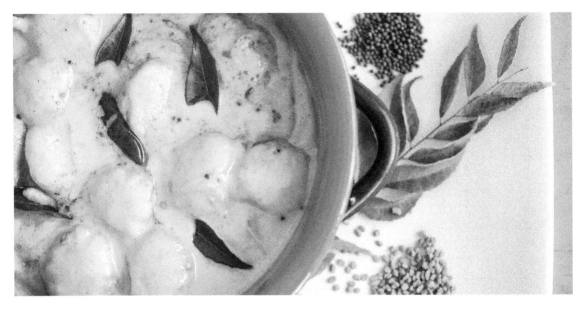

CHICK PEA FLOUR AND YOGURT DISH (KARHI PAKORA)

This dish is bit on the heavy side, perfect for cooler weather in winter or fall and more appropriate for lunch than dinner. Serve with hot chapati, or rice.

- Preparation time: 25 minutes
- Serves 4

Main Ingredients	Herbs/Spices	Oil/Ghee	Kitchen Gear
For Karhi:			
1 cup plain yogurt	½ teaspoon brown mustard seeds	3-4 tablespoons	A large open-
½ cup plus 2 tablespoons	1 teaspoon fenugreek seeds	safflower, coconut,	mouth pan
besan (chick pea flour)	½ teaspoon coriander seeds	or sunflower seed	Blender
4½ cups water	½ teaspoon cumin seeds	oil for the dish	Small kadai or
2-3 green chili peppers cut	4-6 fresh curry leaves		a round- bottom
into long, thin strands	1 teaspoon basic spice mix*	1 teaspoon ghee*	frying pan
1 medium onion cut into long,	½ teaspoon turmeric powder	per serving	Blender
thin strands	¾ teaspoon salt		Perforated
1 tablespoon finely chopped	¼ cup chopped cilantro		cooking spoon
fresh ginger	⅛ teaspoon hing (asafetida)		Plate lined with
	powder		paper towel
	A pinch of black pepper		

Main Ingredients	Herbs/Spices	Oil/Ghee	Kitchen Gear
For Pakoras:			
½ cup besan	¼ teaspoon salt	1-2 cup of safflower, coconut or	
½ cup water	Pinch of black pepper	sunflower seed oil for frying pakoras	

*recipe in Chapter 16

Directions

1. Mix yogurt, besan and 2 cups of water in a blender; set aside.

2. Heat oil in large pan for 15 seconds. Add onions and brown lightly for about 5 minutes. Add chili peppers and ginger to the pan and cook for another minute. Push mixture to the side, allowing oil to settle into the middle of the pan.

3. Add mustard, fenugreek, coriander, cumin seeds and curry leaves. Cook for 15 seconds: the seeds will splutter and brown. Now add the spice mix and turmeric powder, mixing all ingredients together. Add asafetida (hing) to the mixture here.

4. Pour the yogurt mix into the pan, and stir. Put two more cups of water into the blender to get all the batter out and pour into the pan; stir. The liquid will begin to thicken around the edges of the pan, so keep scraping and mixing. Continue to stir until mixture is smooth. If the liquid continues to thicken, add more water a ¼ cup at a time. You don't want it to be too thick or too thin. It should stick to the spoon.

5. Add ¾ teaspoon salt and cook on medium heat for 10-15 minutes, stirring occasionally. If the liquid is sticking too much to the sides of the pan, it is too thick, so add about ½ a cup water. Cover the pan when not stirring, as it will splash and bubble while cooking.

6. Add the pakoras (recipe follows). Turn heat to low and cook for another 10-15 minutes.

7. Garnish with cilantro and a teaspoon of ghee per serving

8. Serve hot and enjoy!

Directions for Pakoras:

1. Heat 2 cups of oil in the round-bottomed pan or kadai for about 5 minutes.

2. In the meantime, using your hands, mix ½ cup of besan with ½ cup of water. Add ¼ teaspoon of salt and a pinch of black pepper. You should be able to pick the mixture up with your hands.

3. Put a tiny drop of the mixture into the pan. If it pops up to the surface, the oil is ready.

4. Take about a tablespoon of the batter into your hands and drop it into the pan taking care not to splash the hot oil. If it seems as though the pakoras are browning too quickly, reduce the heat. When pakoras are brown, scoop them out of the oil with a perforated cooking spoon and drain for a few seconds before placing the pakoras on a plate lined with paper towel. This will absorb the remainder of the oil.

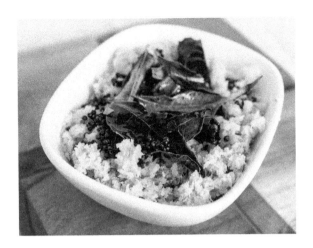

COCONUT CHUTNEY (NARIYAL CHUTNEY)

Traditionally served with South Indian dishes, this can be used with any dish to enhance its digestibility and taste. Great in summer.

- Preparation time: 10 minutes
- Makes 1 cup of chutney

Main Ingredients	Herbs/Spices	Oil/Ghee	Kitchen Gear
1 cup grated coconut ¼ cup chopped cilantro 1 whole red chili pepper 2 green chili peppers, cut in half lengthwise 1 tablespoon chana daal or lentils (optional)	1 teaspoon grated ginger 2-3 tablespoons tamarind, soaked and softened ½ teaspoon brown mustard seeds 4 curry leaves	2 teaspoons oil	Blender Saucepan

Directions

1. Blend coconut, cilantro, chili peppers, chana daal, ginger and tamarind for 5 minutes and pour into a glass container.

2. Heat 2 teaspoons of oil in saucepan for 15 seconds. Add 1 red chili pepper, brown mustard seeds and 3-4 curry leaves. Add this to the chutney, mix it together and refrigerate.

Enjoy!

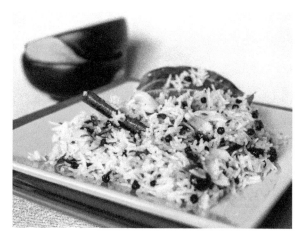

CRANBERRY, BLACK PEPPER, CASHEW RICE

This recipe is from my niece. It is great for gatherings, and holidays, as it has a sweet, spicy and nutty taste.

- Preparation time: 20 minutes
- Serves 4

Main Ingredients	Herbs/Spices	Oil/Ghee	Kitchen Gear
1 cup rice	1 cinnamon stick	2 tablespoons ghee*	Medium bowl
Water	2 bay leaves		Medium frying pan
½ cup cranberries	6 pods green cardamom		Flat spatula
¼ cup cashews	½ teaspoon cumin seeds		Small frying pan
	1 teaspoon salt		
	¼ cup whole peppercorns		

*recipe in Chapter 16

Directions

1. Soak rice in bowl with double the amount of room-temperature water for 10 minutes.
2. Heat ghee in medium pan for a few seconds; add cinnamon stick, bay leaves, cardamom, and cumin seeds.
3. Sauté for 15-20 seconds.
4. Drain the rice then rinse until clear; drain again, then add rice to pan.
5. Use a flat spatula to stir the rice and the spices, taking care not to break the rice.
6. Add 2 cups water, the cranberries and peppercorn.
7. Turn heat to low and cook for 10 minutes.
8. In a separate pan, dry roast the cashews. Add cashews to the rice and mix.

Enjoy!

CUMIN BASMATI RICE (JEERA CHAWAL)

Basmati rice is another household staple in Indian cooking. This makes a great side dish and can be used in combination with other dishes. Basmati rice is light and easy to digest.

- Preparation time: 10 minutes
- Serves 4

Main Ingredients	Herbs/Spices	Oil/Ghee	Kitchen Gear
1 cup long grain basmati rice	1 teaspoon cumin seeds	2 tablespoons oil or ghee*	Medium bowl
1 small onion, thinly sliced (optional)	2-3 whole black cardamoms		Medium frying pan
2 cups water	1 stick cinnamon stick		
	1-2 bay leaves		
	Pinch of salt		

*recipe in Chapter 16

Directions

1. Soak 1 cup long grain basmati rice in bowl in double the amount of lukewarm water for 10-15 minutes.

2. Put ghee or oil in the frying pan and heat on medium for 15 seconds.

3. Add onions (if you are adding them) and cook until light brown.

4. Add cumin, cardamom, cinnamon stick, and bay leaves, and cook for 30 seconds.

5. Drain the water from the rice and rinse two or three times with fresh water, or until the water runs clear. Don't massage the rice as this will break the grains. Drain rice well.

6. Add rice to the spice mixture, stirring it gently until the water dries off. Cook for another minute, add 2 cups water, then stir.

7. When the rice and water begin to boil, turn heat to low and cover the pan, leaving a little space for steam to escape.

8. Cook for 7-10 minutes or until all water is gone. Turn burner off.

9. Remove the lid to prevent the rice from sticking or overcooking.

10. Use a flat spatula to scoop rice from pan to keep grains from breaking.

11. Serve hot with your favorite dish.

Enjoy!

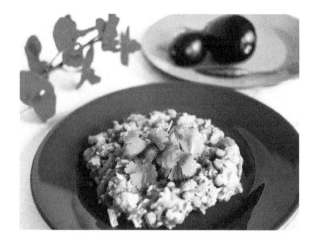

EGGPLANT AND PEAS (BHARTHA)

Eggplant is a nightshade and is heating to our body. But when it is grilled or baked whole, it becomes cooling. This has a smoky flavor and is great for summer. Serve with chapati. It can also be used as a dip with pita chips.

• Preparation time: 20 minutes

• Serves 2-3

Main Ingredients	Herbs/Spices	Oil/Ghee	Kitchen Gear
1 medium eggplant	1 teaspoon cumin seeds	3 tablespoons	Medium bowl
1 medium onion, thinly sliced	1 teaspoon coriander	sunflower oil	Frying pan
1 medium tomato, chopped	seeds	2 teaspoons ghee*	
1 chopped chili	½ teaspoon salt		
½ cup peas	½ teaspoon turmeric		
	½ cup chopped cilantro		

*recipe in Chapter 16

Directions

1. Grill whole eggplant for 20 minutes, turning every few minutes so it cooks evenly. You can also bake in an oven at 325F degrees for 35-40 minutes.

2. Allow eggplant to cool slightly, then peel and put the cooked eggplant in a bowl. Mash well with a fork. There should be no thick parts.

3. Heat oil in pan on medium for 15 seconds, then add onion.

4. Brown the onion, then add tomatoes and chili peppers. Cook for another 2-3 minutes

5. Push the mixture to the side of the pan and then add cumin and coriander. Cook for 15 seconds and then stir, blending spices into the onion and tomato mixture.

6. Stir in the mashed eggplant and salt. Cook on low heat for 15 minutes.

7. Add peas and stir.

8. Garnish with cilantro and ghee.

Enjoy!

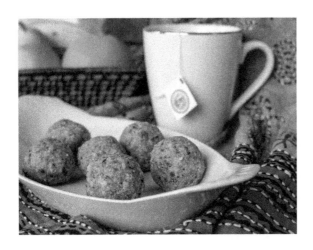

ENERGY BALLS

Great snack to have on hand for quick energy, as a breakfast bar or as a snack with tea.

• Preparation time: 20 minutes

• Makes about 20 small (2") balls

Main Ingredients	Herbs/Spices	Oil/Ghee	Kitchen Gear
1 cup activated barley or soluble rice bran 1 cup chopped dates ½ cup chopped Brazilian nuts ½ cup hemp hearts 2 tablespoons tahini, well-stirred before measuring	½ teaspoon cinnamon ¼ teaspoon cardamom powder 1 teaspoon vanilla Pinch of salt	2 tablespoons coconut oil, melted and divided	Food processor Bowl

Directions

1. Add all ingredients to the bowl and mix. If mixture sticks to the bottom of the bowl, remove it all, knead it manually and return to bowl.

2. Roll dough into balls about 2" across. (You can make these any size you prefer.)

3. Store in a container in the pantry or on your tabletop.

Enjoy!

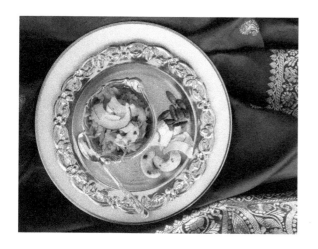

FOUR C'S PUDDING (CARROT, CASHEW, COCONUT, AND CARDAMOM)

A quick and healthy treat. Great as a snack with tea or as a dessert after dinner.

- Preparation time: 15 minutes
- Serves 2-3

Main Ingredients	Herbs/Spices	Oil/Ghee	Kitchen Gear
4 shredded carrots	½ teaspoon whole cardamom seeds	2 tablespoons ghee* or coconut oil	Small pot
⅛ cup water			Small pan
1 tablespoon cane sugar	2 teaspoons coconut pieces		Small bowls
10 cashews			

*recipe in Chapter 16

Directions

1. Heat the ghee in a small pot for 30 seconds and then add cardamom pods and cook for 15 seconds.

2. Add carrots and water. Cook for 10 minutes on slow heat.

3. Turn the heat off and add sugar.

4. Heat up a small pan and dry toast the cashews.

5. Pour into small bowls, then garnish with toasted cashews and coconut.

Enjoy!

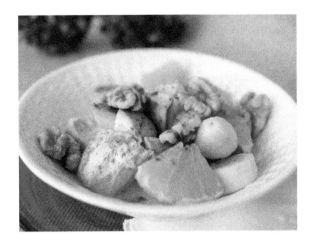

FRUIT AND NUT BOWL

Clear and pure source of energy for the mornings! No guesswork here.

• Preparation time: 5 minutes

• Serves 2

Main Ingredients	Herbs/Spices	Oil/Ghee	Kitchen Gear
¼ cup walnuts	1 teaspoon honey		Medium bowl
1 avocado	Pinch of salt		Paper towel
1 orange	Pinch of Pepper		Small bowl Whisk
1 banana	Pinch of ginger powder		
1/2 lemon			

Directions:

1. Soak walnuts overnight in water.

2. Rinse the walnuts, then clean and dry them on a paper towel.

3. Cut avocado, banana, and orange in small, bite-sized chunks and place in medium bowl.

4. Add the nuts to the fruit bowl.

5. Squeeze lemon juice in a separate bowl. Whisk in 1 teaspoon honey, then add salt, ginger powder and black pepper.

6. Pour over the bowl and stir

Enjoy!

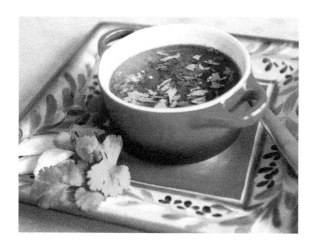

GINGER SOUP (ADARAK KI TARI)

This soup is warming, cleansing and it makes a great digestive aid. Enjoy as an appetizer or as a great healing soup for a cold or the flu.

- Prep time: 15 minutes
- Serves 2-3

Main Ingredients	Herbs/Spices	Oil/Ghee	Kitchen Gear
2 tablespoons shredded ginger	1 teaspoon basic spice mix*	3 teaspoons ghee* or coconut oil	Small pot with lid
½-1 cup green peas, according to your preference	¼ teaspoon turmeric powder		
4 cups water	¼ teaspoon coriander seeds		
¼ cup chopped cilantro or parsley			
½ tomato, finely chopped			

*recipe in Chapter 16

Directions:

1. Put ghee or oil in the pot and heat for 15 seconds on medium. Add basic spice mix, turmeric powder and coriander seeds, then cook, stirring, for 15 seconds.

2. Add ginger and continue to stir for 15-30 seconds, then add tomato and cook for another 30 seconds.

3. Add 4 cups water, cover the pot and bring to a boil. Cook for 10 minutes on medium heat.

4. Add peas and cook for another 2 minutes.

5. Garnish with cilantro or parsley. Serve hot.

Enjoy!

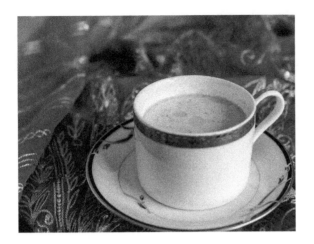

GOLDEN MILK (HALDI KA DHOODH)

Great drink for night time (or any time). It's great as an anti-inflammatory, it's soothing and it's a great sleep aid.

- Preparation time: 5 minutes
- Serves 1

Main Ingredients	Herbs/Spices	Oil/Ghee	Kitchen Gear
1 cup milk* ½ teaspoon honey	½ teaspoon turmeric powder Pepper Saffron	¼ teaspoon ghee**	Small pot

* can substitute with non-dairy milk

** recipe in Chapter 16

Directions

1. Bring milk to boil.
2. Add turmeric powder, honey, and ghee.
3. Turn burner off, pour into a cup and garnish with a touch of black pepper and a few strands of saffron.

Enjoy!

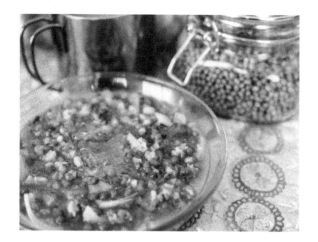

GREEN LENTIL SOUP WITH CELERY (SABUT MUNGI KI DAAL)

This is a nourishing "anytime" recipe. Serve with chapati, rice or as soup. Feel free to add any vegetables that you like here.

- Preparation time: 20 minutes
- Serves 4

Main Ingredients	Herbs/Spices	Oil/Ghee	Kitchen Gear
1 cup whole brown lentils	1 teaspoon cumin	2 tablespoons ghee*	Medium pot
6 cups water	2-3 bay leaves		Small frying pan
1 small onion, sliced thinly (optional)	1 teaspoon grated ginger		
2 stalks celery, cut in small pieces	½ lemon		
	¼ cup chopped cilantro		
	1 teaspoon turmeric		
	1 teaspoon salt		
	Touch of hing		

*recipe in Chapter 16

Directions

1. Soak lentils in warm water in medium pot for 10 minutes. Rinse with fresh water until the water runs clear. Add 6 cups of water and cook on medium heat for 10 minutes.

2. Skim away the white foam that rises to the top. You may have to do this 3-4 times or more, until lentils stop foaming.

3. Turn the heat to low and add celery and bay leaves. Cover pot and let mixture cook for another 5 minutes.

4. Add another ½ cup of water if the soup is too thick. Add salt when the lentils are finished cooking. (Adding salt to uncooked lentils tends to make them hard.)

5. Heat ghee in a small frying pan. Sauté onion until brown, then add all of the spices.

6. Garnish with lemon juice, cilantro and a touch of ghee. Serve hot.

Enjoy!

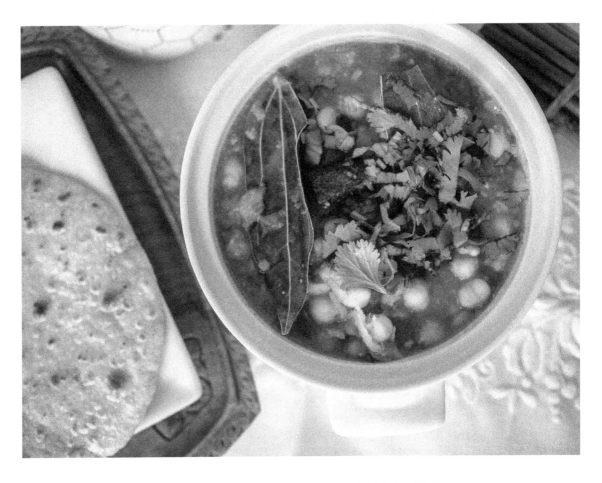

HEARTY SPICED CHICK PEAS (KABULI CHOLLEY)

Serve with rice, bread, or chapati. Good as a soup. You can also add some bitter greens to the dish to make it lighter.

- Preparation time: 20 minutes, plus overnight soak, and minimum 4 hour cooking time for the chick peas

- Serves 6-8

Main Ingredients	Herbs/Spices	Oil/Ghee	Kitchen Gear
2 cups dried chickpeas	3 bay leaves	4-6 teaspoons ghee*	Slow cooker
Water	1 teaspoon cumin seeds	(or oil, if preferred)	Small frying pan
1 small onion, finely chopped	1 teaspoon coriander seeds	(chick peas tend to	Serving spoon
1 tomato, coarsely chopped	2 teaspoons spice mix*	be a little drying, so it	
1 teaspoon grated ginger	1 teaspoon turmeric powder	is good to add extra	
Salt	⅛ teaspoon hing (asafetida)	ghee)	
¼ cup chopped cilantro	1½ teaspoon salt	Small pan	
1-2 green chili peppers	¼ cup chopped fresh cilantro		
chopped (optional)			

* recipe in Chapter 16

Directions:

1. Soak chickpeas in 8 times their volume of warm water overnight in the slow cooker.

2. Rinse well with fresh water. Drain all water out of the slow cooker and add 8 cups fresh water plus the bay leaves.

3. Plug the slow cooker in and place on high heat. Set timer for at least 4 hours and up to 8 hours. (For some slow cookers 4 hours is sufficient time.)

4. When timer sounds, check the chickpeas to see if they are soft. Turn the slow cooker to warm.

5. With a serving spoon, mash some of the chick peas by pressing them to the side of the cooker to thicken the soup a little.

6. Heat ghee/oil in a small pan for 15 seconds, and then add onions, browning slightly.

7. Add tomatoes and ginger once the onions are light brown. Add a touch of salt. Let this cook for 3-5 minutes on medium heat.

8. Push the mixture to the side and allow ghee to pool in the bottom of the pan. Add cumin and coriander seeds first, and then add the spice mix, turmeric powder, hing powder. Mix and cook for another minute.

9. Add this mixture to the slow cooker. Add salt and mix.

10. Garnish with cilantro and a drizzle of ghee.

11. Serve hot.

Enjoy!

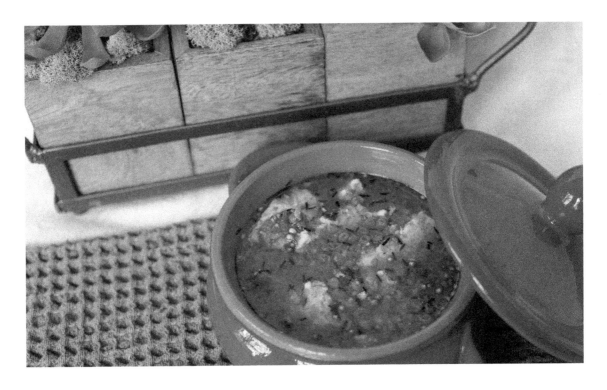

HOMEMADE CHEESE AND PEA CURRY (MUTTER PANEER)

This is bit on the rich and heavy side. This dish is hearty, satisfying and simply delicious. It is a treat! Paneer is homemade cheese, which is highly nutritious. Serve with rice or chapati. The homemade cheese is fresher and easier to digest than commercially available cheeses.

- Preparation time: 30 minutes
- Serves 4-5

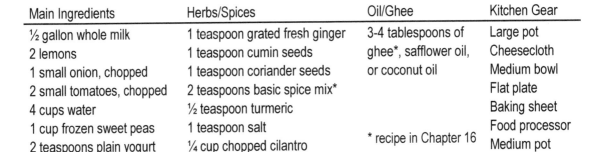

Main Ingredients	Herbs/Spices	Oil/Ghee	Kitchen Gear
½ gallon whole milk	1 teaspoon grated fresh ginger	3-4 tablespoons of	Large pot
2 lemons	1 teaspoon cumin seeds	ghee*, safflower oil,	Cheesecloth
1 small onion, chopped	1 teaspoon coriander seeds	or coconut oil	Medium bowl
2 small tomatoes, chopped	2 teaspoons basic spice mix*		Flat plate
4 cups water	½ teaspoon turmeric		Baking sheet
1 cup frozen sweet peas	1 teaspoon salt		Food processor
2 teaspoons plain yogurt	¼ cup chopped cilantro	* recipe in Chapter 16	Medium pot

Directions for Paneer

1. Pour milk into the large pot, bring it to a boil, then turn off the heat.

2. Juice one lemon and stir it into the milk. If solids begin to form, you don't need more lemon. If this does not happen, turn the heat back on to medium and add the juice from half of another lemon. This may take 2-3 minutes. Keep stirring.

3. Strain the liquid through a piece of cheesecloth draped across the top of a bowl. Allow excess liquid to fully drain into the bowl and then fold cheesecloth into a little pouch. Place the pouch on a flat plate, flatten it with your hands, and put a heavy pot on top of it so the cheese can settle. Set aside for 30 minutes.

4. Preheat oven to 175-200F degrees. Cut cheese into small squares and place them on a greased baking sheet; bake in the oven for 7-10 minutes.

Directions for Curried Peas

1. Put chopped onions in the food processor and pulse until finely minced.

2. Add ghee/oil to the medium pot and heat for 15 seconds, then add onions and cook for 2-4 minutes until they brown.

3. In the meantime, put tomatoes in the food processor and pulse until finely minced. And add them to the pot once the onions are browned.

4. Add ginger and cook the whole mixture for another 5 minutes on low heat.

5. Move this mixture to the side of the pot and allow the remaining oil to pool in the bottom of the pot. Add cumin, coriander, spice mix, turmeric and salt to the oil, and let them cook for 1 minute.

6. Add yogurt and mix all ingredients.

7. Add 4 cups of water, cover the pot and let mixture cook for 10 minutes on medium heat.

8. Remove paneer from oven, add to pot and cook on low heat for another 5 minutes.

9. Rinse the frozen peas in tap water and add to the pot. Cook for another 5 minutes on low heat.

10. Turn the heat off and serve hot.

11. Garnish with cilantro

Enjoy!

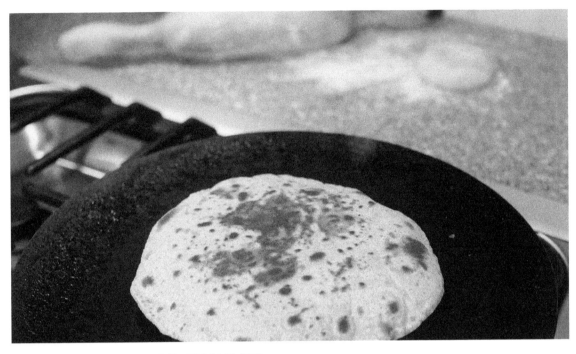

INDIAN FLAT BREAD (CHAPATI)

Chapati is a staple in Indian kitchens and is prepared fresh at each meal. It is very versatile, and can be eaten with meals or plain as a snack with just butter and salt, like toast. The only ingredients are water and flour. The dough can be made right when you need it. But it is better to make it ahead of time and cover it with a wet dish cloth for at least half hour before cooking so it does not dry out.

- Preparation time: 20 minutes
- Makes 3 chapatis

Main Ingredients	Herbs/Spices	Oil/Ghee	Kitchen Gear
1 cup chapati flour*			Large bowl
1/2 cup water			Tawa **
			Rolling pin
			Paper towel
			Dish towel

*Available at Indian grocery stores. **Tawa is a flat disc shape frying pan to make chapati. You can improvise by just using a non-stick frying pan

Directions

1. Put flour in a large bowl.
2. Add water and stir with your hands until dough forms. You may need another teaspoon of water to mix all the flour.
3. Knead the dough with your hands until smooth.
4. Cover the bowl with a lid or a wet paper towel and set it aside for 30 minutes.
5. Knead dough again for 1 minute.
6. Heat the tawa on medium heat.
7. Take a small piece of dough, toss it in dry flour and roll it into a small, smooth ball between your palms.
8. Flatten the ball with your hands and roll it in some dry flour again.
9. Place the flattened ball on countertop or a wooden board and roll it into a circle.
10. You may need to sprinkle a little dry flour on the surface if the chapati begins to stick, or simply pick it up and toss it in the dry flour again. Finished chapati should be about 6" in diameter.
11. Pick chapati up and toss it from hand to hand, whipping some air into it. This will make sure that it is light when cooked.
12. Drop a little dough on the tawa. If it burns too quickly, turn the heat to low. If it begins to just brown, the tawa is ready. Put the chapati on the pan and cook for about 30 seconds. Flip it over and leave it on this side longer, frequently shifting it to make sure the entire surface gets cooked.
13. Flip chapati over again and now gently press it with a dish towel. You don't want to smush it down, just gently coax it to balloon up.
14. Remove from heat, butter the chapati and serve hot.

Enjoy!

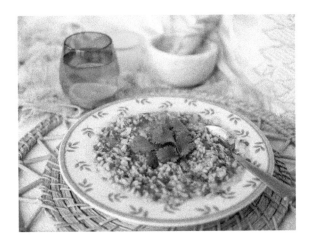

LENTIL AND RICE SOUP (KHICHARHI)

Khicharhi is a potent blood purifier and also supports proper kidney function. It's great for spring, and it's a go-to dish whenever there is nothing else around to eat. It's also ideal when you are not feeling well and want to eat light.

• Preparation time: 20 minutes

• Serves 3-4

Main Ingredients	Herbs/Spices	Oil/Ghee	Kitchen Gear
½ cup white basmati rice	½ teaspoon fresh grated ginger	2 tablespoons ghee**	Medium pot
1 cup split yellow mung beans (or any type of lentil), or just use 1 cup khicharhi mix*	¼ - ½ teaspoon salt		Small frying pan
	¼ teaspoon mustard seeds (optional)		
4 cups water	¼ teaspoon fenugreek seeds (optional)		
	¼ teaspoon cumin seeds (optional)		
	Pinch of hing (asafetida)		
*available in Indian grocery stores	1 teaspoon Spice Mix**		
	Fresh cilantro		

** recipe in Chapter 16

Directions

1. Soak rice and lentils or khicharhi mix in warm water in medium pot for 5-10 minutes. Rinse rice and lentils until the water runs clear.

2. Add 4 cups of water to the pot and cook on medium heat for 10-15 minutes. Skim off the white foam. You may have to do this a few times.

3. Reduce heat and continue cooking for another 5-10 minutes or until the ingredients are soft. Add more water if mixture starts to dry out; then add enough water (½ to 1 cup) to ensure mixture is the consistency of soup. Add ginger and salt.

4. In a separate pan, heat ghee for 15 seconds. Add all whole seed spices and stir for 20 seconds. When the seeds begin to cook, add ½ - 1 teaspoon of spice mix. Cook for one minute.

5. Garnish with cilantro and a little bit of ghee.

Enjoy!

MINT CHUTNEY (PUDEENE KI CHUTNEY)

A great digestive aid; good with any meal.

- Preparation time: 5 minutes
- Makes little bit more than 1 cup

Main Ingredients	Herbs/Spices	Oil/Ghee	Kitchen Gear
¼ cup tamarind pulp or juice of 1 lemon 2 bunches mint leaves, washed 4 whole green onions or 1 small onion 2-3 green chili peppers Lemon juice	1 teaspoon grated ginger 1 teaspoon roasted cumin seeds ¼ teaspoon sugar ½ teaspoon salt 2 teaspoons pomegranate seeds ¼ teaspoon turbinado		Small frying pan Blender

Directions

1. Soak tamarind pulp (if you are using it) in 1/2 cup of warm water for one hour. Mash it up with your hands, remove any hard bits. Set aside.

2. Heat small pan on high heat for 2 minutes. Add cumin seeds and turn the heat off. Shake the pan slightly so the seeds roast evenly.

3. Add hydrated tamarind pulp or lemon juice, mint leaves, onions, chili peppers, and ginger to blender and purée. Add cumin seeds, sugar, salt, pomegranate seeds and blend for another minute

4. Store in a glass jar and refrigerate. Keeps for 2-3 weeks

Enjoy with meals as a digestive aid.

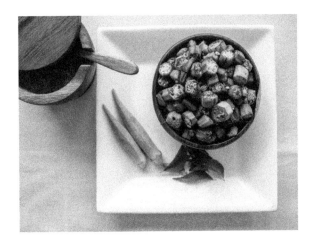

OKRA (BHINDI)

Okra is a special vegetable that needs to be washed and cooked dry without any water. Makes a great side dish with a lentil soup; serve with chapati.

- Preparation time: 20 minutes
- Serves 2-3

Main Ingredients	Herbs/Spices	Oil/Ghee	Kitchen Gear
½ lb. Okra	½ teaspoon cumin seeds 1 teaspoon spice mix* ¼ teaspoon salt	2 tablespoons coconut oil or safflower oil	Paper towel Medium frying pan

* recipe in Chapter 16

Directions

1. Wash okra thoroughly and lay on a paper towel to dry.

2. Lay another paper towel on top of the okra and roll gently to dry thoroughly. Ensure the okra is completely dry.

3. Cut off and discard the tops and bottoms of each piece of okra, then cut remaining okra into small pieces. Take care to ensure your knife and hands remain dry throughout this process.

4. Add oil to frying pan and heat on medium heat for 15-20 seconds.

5. Add cumin seeds and spice mix and cook for 15 seconds.

6. Add okra and salt and stir (okra should be completely dry, as any water will make it slimy)

7. Lower heat slightly and cover the pot with lid that has been flipped upside down. Add one teaspoon of water to the lid. (This is a condensation technique that drips just a little water at a time into the pot to ensure the okra does not burn, as there is no water in the pan at the start of the cooking process.)

8. Cook for about 10 minutes and then check to see if the okra is soft.

Serve with a side dish or chapati and enjoy!

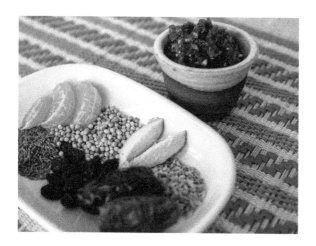

RAISIN DATE CHUTNEY

This is great to have around in the fridge as a sweet little-pick-me-up snack, or you can put it on toast or crackers and eat with meals.

• Preparation time: 10 minutes

• Makes 2 cups of chutney

Main Ingredients	Herbs/Spices	Oil/Ghee	Kitchen Gear
1 ½ cups raisins	1 ½ teaspoons fennel seeds		2 medium bowls
¾ cup dates, pitted and chopped	1 ½ teaspoons cumin seeds		Paper towel
⅜ cup orange juice	3 teaspoons coriander seeds		Small pan
	⅜ teaspoon salt		Mortar and pestle
	¼ teaspoon ground nutmeg		Food processor
	2 tablespoons fresh ginger, minced		Glass container with lid

Directions

1. Place dates and raisins in separate bowls, cover with water, and soak for an hour

2. Rinse and drain well and lay on a paper towel to dry.

3. Remove pits from the dates and chop them into small chunks.

4. Put a small pan on the stove on high heat for 2 minutes. Put fennel, cumin, and coriander seeds in the pan, stirring the pan a little to roast evenly—you will begin to smell when they are roasted. Coarsely grind them manually with a mortar and pestle.

5. Place the dates, raisins, and spices into the food processer and add the orange juice

6. Pulse in food processor until everything is coarsely ground. If the mixer looks too thick and does not move, add a couple of teaspoons of orange juice.

7. Add salt, nutmeg, and ginger, and pulse again briefly.

8. Pour into a glass container and refrigerate.

Enjoy with meals or by itself.

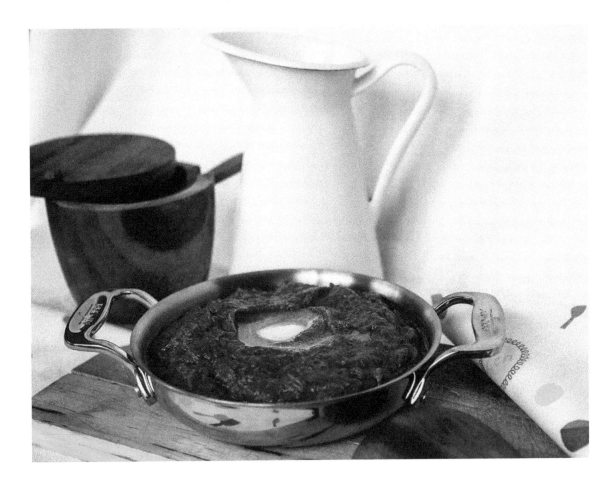

RAPINI AND BROCCOLI SAAG (SARSAUN KA SAAG)

A great dish anytime and can be made with any greens of your choice. Rapini Saag is very typical in Northern India and is served with yellow corn bread. If you are cooking for one, as I often am, I will freeze part of this to be used within a week or two. You can sauté it with fresh onions, tomatoes and ginger to liven it up—it tastes yummy! This dish is best enjoyed with chapati or any other flat bread. As bitter greens can be drying, serving them with a little extra ghee is always nice...and tastes great!

- Prep time: 25 minutes
- Serves 2-3

Main Ingredients	Herbs/Spices	Oil/Ghee	Kitchen Gear
1 bunch fresh rapini, chopped coarsely ½ cup water, more if necessary 1 stalk broccoli ½ small tomato, chopped ½ small onion 1 teaspoon chopped ginger ½ small chili (optional)	½ teaspoon fenugreek seeds ½ teaspoon salt 1 teaspoon chick pea flour or arrowroot flour for binding or thickening.	3-4 teaspoons ghee*	Colander Medium pot Hand blender, food processor or blender Small frying pan

* recipe in Chapter 16

Directions

1. Place rapini in the colander and give it a good wash.

2. Transfer it to the pot, add ½ cup of water, cover the pot and put it on the stove on medium heat.

3. Cook for 10 minutes, checking every few minutes to make sure it does not dry out. If it does, add another ½ cup of water.

4. Wash the broccoli, chop it in small pieces (include the stem and leaves) and add to the pot. Keep the pot covered.

5. Cook for another 10 minutes. There should be no water remaining in the pot. Turn the stove off.

6. Use a hand blender to blend the mixture in the pot, or put the mixture in a blender or food processor to purée.

7. Transfer puréed vegetables back to the pot if they were not puréed there.

8. Mix chick pea flour or the other thickener in a little bit of water and add it to the pot.

9. Turn the heat to low, add salt and cook for another 5 minutes, stirring occasionally.

10. In a separate pan, heat ghee and then sauté onions until brown. Add tomato and ginger and cook for another 2 minutes.

11. Push the mix to the side and add fenugreek seeds. Cook for 15 seconds, and then add to the main pot and stir.

12. Garnish with ghee.

Enjoy!

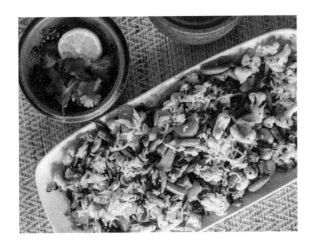

RICE WITH VEGETABLES AND NUTS

Another great Sunday Brunch idea! Add your choice of vegetables. You can make rice at the same time so both the vegetables and rice get done at the same time. My favorites are cauliflower, carrots, green beans, and peas. Serve with mint or coconut chutney.

• Preparation time 30 minutes

• Serves 2-3

Main Ingredients	Herbs/Spices	Oil/Ghee	Kitchen/Gear
¼ cup chopped onion	1 tablespoon brown mustard seeds	3 tablespoons safflower oil, olive oil or coconut oil	Medium pan Small frying pan
1 small potato, chopped	1 teaspoon cumin seeds		
1 cup chopped beans	5-6 curry leaves		
1 cup chopped cauliflower	2 green chili peppers, chopped		
½ cup chopped carrots	½ teaspoon turmeric powder		
½ cup frozen peas	2 lemons		
½ cup peanuts or cashews	½ cup chopped cilantro		
2 cups cooked rice	1 teaspoon salt		
	Dash of black pepper		

Directions

1. Put oil in pan and heat for 1-2 minutes.

2. Add onion and sauté until light brown. Push onion aside and let the oil pool in the bottom of the pan. Then add mustard seeds, cumin seeds, curry leaves, chili peppers and turmeric powder. Stir and then add all veggies, plus the salt and pepper. Cover and cook for 7-10 minutes on slightly less-than-medium heat.

3. Once the vegetables are cooked, turn the heat off.

4. Dry roast the peanuts or cashews in small frying pan and add to the mixture.

5. Add 2 cups of cooked rice to the mixture, mix it well and cover the pan for 2 minutes to let the flavor to infuse together.

6. Garnish with cilantro.

Enjoy!

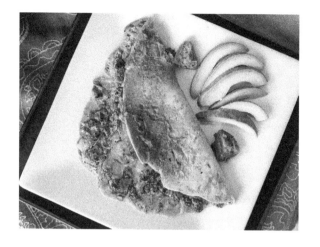

SAVORY CHICK PEA PANCAKE (BESAN KA PURAH)

Chick pea flour is versatile and this particular recipe is great for a Sunday Brunch! Packed with nutrition and tasty, you may make this plain and eat it with a vegetable dish or add the vegetables I've suggested here right into the pancake.

- Preparation time: 10 minutes
- Serves 2

Main Ingredients	Herbs/Spices	Oil/Ghee	Kitchen Gear
½ cup besan (chick pea flour)	¼ teaspoon celery seeds	4 teaspoons of ghee* or butter	Blender
½ cup water	¼ teaspoon coriander seeds		Non-stick pan
1 teaspoon semolina or cream of wheat	A little less than ¼ teaspoon salt		
¼ onion, cut in thin small slices			
Handful of spinach, chopped			
¼ cup chopped cilantro			

* recipe in Chapter 16

Directions

1. Mix besan and water in a blender or vita mix to a smooth consistency.
2. Add semolina or cream of wheat and mix with a fork.
3. Add onion, spinach, cilantro and all of the spices.
4. The mixture should be the consistency of pancake batter. You may need to add a bit more water to thin it out if it is too thick.
5. Heat a nonstick pan on medium heat for one minute.
6. Pour mixture into pan and gently spread with a wooden spatula. No need to grease the pan.
7. Cook for 3-4 minutes or until the edges begin to lift off of the pan.
8. Gently flip the purah over and cook the other side for another 3-4 minutes
9. Turn off heat. Slide purah onto your plate, and spread surface with 2 teaspoons of ghee or butter
10. Serve with avocado.

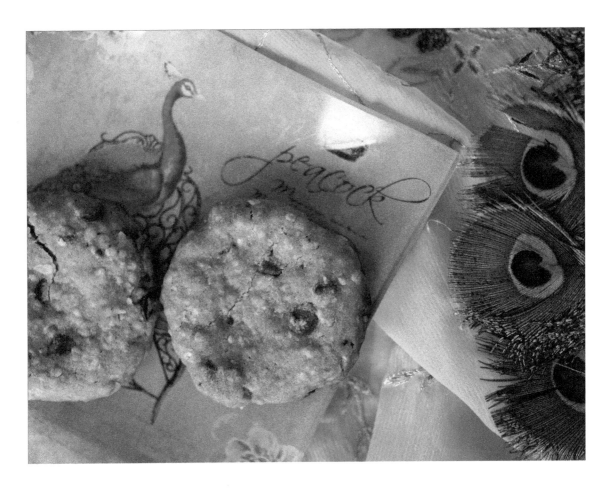

SMART COOKIES

I never baked until I became a mom. I got this recipe for chocolate chip cookies in the mail on a card from Great American Home Baking. I followed the recipe, as I have no skills when it comes to baking. These became my son's favorite cookies and we bake them on special occasions and "just because." When my son left home to go to college, I started to sneak healthier ingredients into the recipe and that's how these "smart cookies" were invented. Yup! Cookies! Mom's secret weapon!

- Preparation time: 20 minutes
- Makes 30-40 cookies

Main Ingredients	Herbs/Spices	Oil/Ghee	Kitchen Gear
1 cup all-purpose flour	1 tablespoon aluminum-free	2.5 sticks unsalted	Medium mixing bowl
1 cup almond meal	baking powder	butter, softened	Large mixing bowl
½ cup coconut sugar	1 tablespoon cinnamon		Hand mixer
¼ cup turbinado sugar	powder		Plastic wrap
1 large egg	1 tablespoon vanilla extract		Cookie sheet
1 cup carob chips			
1 cup oats			

Directions

1. Remove butter from fridge two hours prior to making cookies to soften.
2. Preheat oven to 300F degrees.
3. Sift all-purpose flour into a mixing bowl.
4. Add almond meal, baking powder, and cinnamon, and mix well.
5. In a separate bowl, beat butter, turbinado sugar, and coconut sugar together at medium speed until light and fluffy.
6. Beat in egg and vanilla extract.
7. Mix flour in at low speed until blended. Scrape dough off beaters.
8. Mix oats and carob chips into the dough with your hands.
9. Cover with plastic wrap and chill for one hour.
10. Shape dough into small balls (about 2" in diameter) and place on ungreased baking sheet. Flatten them with the palm of your hand and put the baking sheet into the oven.
11. Bake until lightly brown, 10-12 minutes. Check partway through to avoid burning the cookies, as oven temperatures are not consistent. Remove from oven and transfer to a cooling rack or a plate to cool for about 5 minutes before serving.

Enjoy!

Want fresh cookies at the drop of a hat?

Make small cookie logs about 6" long and 2" thick, and wrap them individually in wax paper. Place them in a plastic bag and freeze. You can take one log out and bake cookies whenever you want fresh, warm cookies. Each log will make 5-6 cookies.

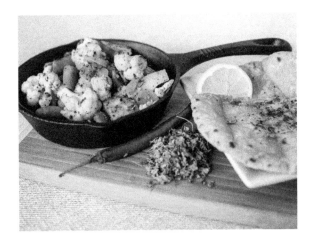

SPICED MIXED VEGETABLES (SABJI)

Great as a side dish Serve with chapati, rice or bread

• Preparation time: 20 minutes

• Serves 2

Main Ingredients	Herbs/Spices	Oil/Ghee	Kitchen Gear
1 small potato - cut into small chunks ½ cup chopped carrots 2 cups chopped cauliflower 1 cup pea pods (cut in half) or green beans	1 teaspoon brown mustard seeds ½ teaspoon cumin seeds ½ teaspoon turmeric powder ¼ teaspoon ginger powder 1 teaspoon basic spice mix (optional)* ½ -1 teaspoon salt Dash of black pepper ¼ cup chopped cilantro or fresh basil 2 teaspoons chopped dill	2 tablespoons ghee* or Coconut Oil	Medium pan with lid

* recipe in Chapter 1

Directions

1. Put oil/ghee in frying pan and heat on medium for 15 seconds

2. Add mustard and cumin seeds, followed 15 seconds later by turmeric powder, ginger powder and basic spice mix, if using. Mix.

3. Add potatoes and mix it into the spices. Add 2 teaspoons of water and cover the pot. Cook on medium heat for 5 minutes. (We add potatoes first as they take longer to cook)

4. Add remaining vegetables, and the salt and pepper. Mix gently, cover the pan, and cook for another 5 minutes.

5. Check to make sure that the vegetables are not sticking to the pan. If they are, turn the heat to low and add a teaspoon of water to the pan, and cook for another 5 minutes.

6. Garnish with cilantro or basil or dill.

Enjoy!

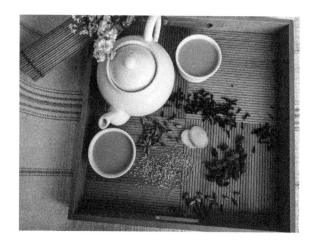

SPICED TEA (MASALA CHAI)

Rich, aromatic comfort in the mornings. Great for sharing in late afternoon. You can always leave out the black tea to eliminate caffeine.

• Preparation time: 10 minutes

• Makes 2 cups

Main Ingredients	Herbs/Spices	Oil/Ghee	Kitchen Gear
2 Cups Water	2 tablespoons fennel seeds		Spice grinder
1 teaspoon loose black tea	1 tablespoon cloves		Small pot
¼ cup milk	3 sticks of cinnamon		Small strainer
	1 teaspoon green cardamom		
	5 black cardamom – if available		
	Licorice		
	2-3 slices fresh ginger		

Directions

1. Grind spices together and store in a glass jar.

2. Put water, 2-3 slices of fresh ginger root, and 1 teaspoon of the chai spice mix in to a small pot and bring to a boil on medium heat. Turn the heat down and let it simmer for another 2 minutes.

3. Add milk and boil for another 2-3 minutes.

4. Add black tea and turn the heat off. If you would like a stronger chai, you can let it boil for another 2 minutes and/or add more black tea

5. Use a small strainer to pour tea into cups. Add honey or sugar to taste.

Enjoy with vegetable fritters (pakoras) or by itself.

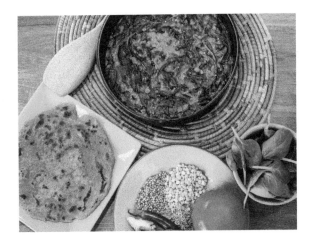

SPINACH WITH LENTILS (DAAL PAALAK)

This protein-rich dish is very filling and satisfying. Enjoy with salad, chapati or rice.

- Preparation time: 20 minutes
- Serves 2

Main Ingredients	Herbs/Spices	Oil/Ghee	Kitchen Gear
1 cup yellow chana daal 4 cups water 3-4 handfuls spinach 1 small onion cut into long thin strands ½ tomato chopped coarsely	1 teaspoon finely chopped ginger ½ teaspoon coriander seeds ½ teaspoon cumin seeds 1 teaspoon spice mix* ½ teaspoon salt	3-4 tablespoons ghee*	Medium pot Potato masher Small frying pan

*recipe in Chapter 16

Directions

1. Soak daal in warm water in medium pot for 10-15 minutes. Rinse with water until clear.

2. Add 4 cups of water and bring to a boil, skimming and discarding the white foam that builds up as daal cooks. Reduce the heat to a little less than medium. Cover the pot, leaving a little gap for steam to escape. Cook for another 10 minutes.

3. Check the daal. It should be soft enough to squish with your fingers. Mash gently with a potato masher 2-3 times.

4. To prepare the Tarka, heat ghee and sauté onion in a separate pan. When onion is light brown, add ginger and tomato, and cook for another 3-5 minutes.

5. Push the ingredients in the pan to one side and allow the remaining ghee to pool in the middle. Add all the spices to the ghee and cook for 15 seconds

6. Tear spinach into small pieces and add to the pan. Cook for 2-3 minutes and add the daal mixture to the pan; mix.

7. Cook together for another 2 minutes on medium heat.

8. Top with a teaspoon of ghee.

Serve hot. Enjoy!

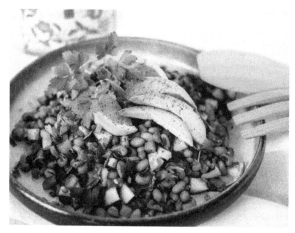

SPRING BLACK EYED PEA SALAD

This has become my favorite summer salad. It is light, vibrant and has all six tastes. Enjoy as a side dish or by itself.

• Prep time: 20 minutes

• Serves 4

Main Ingredients	Herbs/Spices	Oil/Ghee	Kitchen Gear
1 cup black-eyed peas	½ teaspoon cumin seeds	2 teaspoons ghee*	Medium pot
4 cups water plus more for soaking	A pinch of asafetida (hing)	or olive oil	Small frying
small red, orange and yellow sweet	½ teaspoon basic spice mix*	2 teaspoons olive	pan
peppers (2 of each)	½ lemon	oil or avocado oil	
½ red onion	½ teaspoon salt		
2 stalks of celery	Dash of pepper		
¼ small cucumber	Dash of salt		
1 cup chopped parsley	1 teaspoon capers		
1 small green chili (optional)	2-3 slices of avocado (optional)		*recipe in Chapter 16

Directions

1. Soak black eyed peas in a medium pot in at least two cups water overnight, if possible, but for at least one hour before cooking. Rinse peas in water until clear, then add 4 cups of water and bring to a boil on medium heat; boil for 10 minutes.

2. Skim off the white foam that develops and discard. You may have to do this 2-3 times until no additional foam appears. Reduce heat to low, cover pot and cook for another 5 minutes. Check to make sure that the peas are soft before turning the heat off.

3. In a small pan, heat ghee for 15 seconds, add all spices and let cook for 15 seconds; add mixture to the peas.

4. Cut vegetables into small chunks and place in a large bowl, then add a dash of black pepper and a pinch of salt.

5. Add lemon and oil (olive or avocado) and mix well.

6. Beans should be piping hot by now. Drain and add to the vegetables. Mix.

7. Garnish with a few slices of avocado, a sliver of lemon and a twig of parsley.

Enjoy!

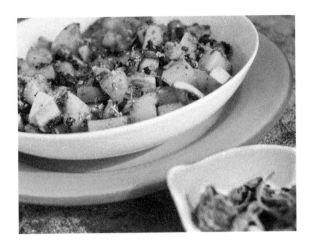

STOVE TOP ACORN SQUASH (KADDU)

I find that cooking on a stove top takes less time than cooking in an oven and I can control the temperature better. The texture of most food cooked this way is also much better, as baking can make some foods— like acorn squash—too soft. You can take the peels off if you like before cutting it into pieces. Leaving the peel on makes this a little crunchy, but with a soft inside.

• Preparation time: 20 minutes

• Serves 4

Main Ingredients	Herbs/Spices	Oil/Ghee	Kitchen Gear
1 small onion, diced 1 small acorn squash, cut into squares, with skin	1 tablespoon fenugreek seeds 1 teaspoon mustard seeds ½ teaspoon salt 2 tablespoons crushed sage leaves 1 tablespoon coconut flakes ½ teaspoon turmeric ¼ teaspoon ginger powder	4 tablespoons coconut or safflower oil	Medium pan with lid

Directions

1. Heat oil in frying pan, then add onion.

2. Brown onion and then add fenugreek and mustard seeds. Cook for 30 seconds, and then add turmeric, ginger powder, and half the sage leaves.

3. Add squash, salt, and water. Turn the lid over and add a few drops of water to it to ensure ingredients do not burn. Let cook for 5-10 minutes on medium heat, checking every few minutes for signs of burning.

4. Remove from heat and serve; garnish with some sage and coconut flakes.

Enjoy as a side dish.

TAMARIND SWEET AND SOUR CHUTNEY (IMLEE KI CHUTNEY)

A great digestive aid; good with any meal, but especially good with vegetable fritters (pakorahs)

• Preparation time: 10 minutes plus one hour for soaking tamarind
• Makes about cup and a half

Main Ingredients	Herbs/Spices	Oil/Ghee	Kitchen Gear
½ cup tamarind, seeded	2 tablespoons cane sugar		Small frying pan
	1 teaspoon cumin seeds		Spice grinder
	½ teaspoon salt		Mortar and pestle
	¼ teaspoon black pepper		Strainer
	¼ teaspoon mango powder		Small Bowl
	A dash of ginger powder		
	A dash of red chili powder		

Directions

1. Run the tamarind under warm water to rinse it off and then soak it in a cup of warm water for an hour.
2. Mesh it together with your hands so all the peaces are dissolved in water. You may have to add another 1/4 cup of water here.
3. Take out any hard peaces or seeds with your hands.
4. Strain the rest of the mixture with a strainer into a small bowl.
5. Heat small pan on high heat for 2 minutes. Add cumin seeds and turn the heat off. Shake the pan slightly so the seeds roast evenly. Coarsely grind the cumin seeds with mortar and pestle.
6. Put the sugar in the spice grinder so it is powdered and can easily dissolve.
7. Add all the spices, sugar and cumin powder to the bowl, mixing it gently.
8. Serve fresh with the fritters and store the remainder in a glass jar and refrigerate. Keeps for 2-3 weeks

Enjoy !

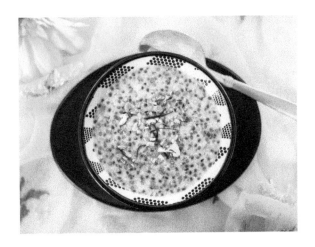

TAPIOCA, CHIA, HEMP SEED PUDDING

This is a great recipe for a healthy sweet snack. It can also be enjoyed for breakfast or as a dessert.

• Preparation time: 15 minutes

• Serves 3-4

Main Ingredients	Herbs/Spices	Oil/Ghee	Kitchen Gear
¼ cup tapioca	¼ teaspoon cardamom powder		Small bowls
¼ cup chia seeds	2 teaspoons rose water		Medium pot
1 cup water	A few strands saffron		
1½ cups whole milk*			
¼ cup hemp seeds			
4 dates			
1 teaspoon chopped pistachios			

*non-dairy substitute may be used

Directions

1. Put tapioca seeds in one cup of water, and let sit for 10 minutes.

2. Place chia seeds in ½ cup of water and let sit for 10 minutes.

3. Bring milk to a boil in medium pot.

4. Drain water from tapioca seeds and add to milk; add chia seeds to milk. (Chia seeds will have expanded in the water and can't be drained).

5. Cook for 5 minutes on low heat.

6. Turn the heat off and add hemp seeds.

7. Stir in rose water.

8. Chop dates into small pieces and add to mixture.

9. Garnish with cardamom powder, a few threads of saffron and the chopped pistachios.

10. Serve warm or chilled.

Enjoy!

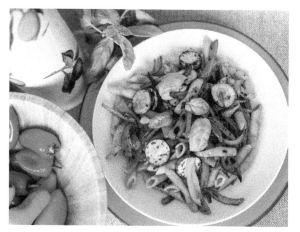

TURMERIC PASTA WITH PAN-GRILLED VEGETABLES

This is a tasty summer meal and a great way to enjoy fresh vegetables. It is not too heavy, and can be enjoyed for both lunch and dinner.

- Preparation time: 20 minutes
- Serves 2

Main Ingredients	Herbs/Spices	Oil/Ghee	Kitchen Gear
6 cups water	½ teaspoon rosemary	1 teaspoon	Medium pot
1 cup whole wheat penne pasta	½ teaspoon fenugreek or basil leaves	olive oil	Large bowl
1 small onion cut in big pieces	⅛ teaspoon powdered ginger	2 teaspoons	Large frying
½ zucchini, sliced	⅛ teaspoon black pepper	safflower oil	pan Medium
8 small colored peppers, diced in	2 cloves garlic, minced		frying pan
big chunks	¼ cup chopped fresh basil leaves		
1 small peeled tomato, halved and	½ teaspoon salt		
shredded	½ teaspoon turmeric		

Directions

1. Put 6 cups of water into a pot and add 1 teaspoon of olive oil (the oil will prevent the pasta from sticking.) Bring the water to a boil (takes about 5 minutes.). Add pasta to the pot and give it a quick stir. Turn the heat to medium and let it cook for 10 minutes.

2. While pasta is cooking, toss onions, peppers, and zucchini together in a bowl, along with the safflower oil, rosemary, fenugreek or basil leaves, ginger, black pepper, and salt. Let the mixture sit for 10 minutes.

3. Strain cooked pasta, rinse it with cold water; set aside.

4. Heat a teaspoon of olive oil in the medium frying pan 15 seconds on medium heat. Add garlic, basil, and turmeric. Cook for 30 seconds. Add the shredded tomato and salt. Cook for 2-3 minutes on low heat. Add pasta to the mixture and cook for one minute.

5. Preheat large frying pan for 3-5 minutes on medium heat. Add the marinaded vegetables. Toss gently to make sure they are cooking evenly for about 2 minutes. You may need to turn the heat down a little to avoid burning the vegetables.

6. Mix the vegetables with the pasta mixture. Serve hot with a little drizzle of olive oil.

Enjoy!

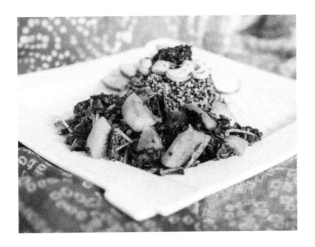

TURNIPS WITH SPINACH (PAALAK SHALGUM)

This is a light and bitter dish that's great as a side.

- Preparation time: 20 minutes
- Serves 2

Main Ingredients	Herbs/Spices	Oil/Ghee	Kitchen Gear
4 turnips 4 handfuls of spinach or baby kale	½ teaspoon fenugreek seeds ½ teaspoon turmeric powder ½ teaspoon grated ginger ¼ teaspoon salt	2 teaspoons ghee*	I medium frying pan with lid Potato masher
			*recipe in Chapter 16

Directions

1. Peel turnips and cut in small 1" cubes.
2. Add ghee to pan and heat for 15 seconds.
3. Add fenugreek seeds and cook for 15 seconds, then add turmeric and ginger.
4. Add turnips and cover the pan.
5. Let cook for 10 minutes, checking to see if the dish is becoming too dry. If it is, add 1 teaspoon of water.
6. Add spinach and cook for another 5 minutes.
7. Gently mash all ingredients. Serve with any grain or some chapati

Enjoy!

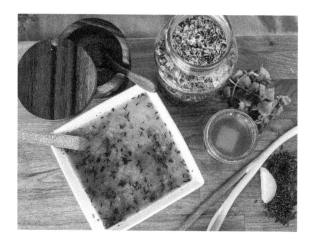

YELLOW LENTILS (MUNGI KI DAAL)

This is another staple for dinners at Indian households due to its lightness. It's easy to digest and tasty and it's a good companion to rice or chapati. Makes a great base for soups and you can add vegetables to make it more hearty. Add the vegetables once the daal (lentil base) has been brought to a boil and all foam has been removed.

- Preparation time: 20 minutes
- Serves 4

Main Ingredients	Herbs/Spices	Oil/Ghee	Kitchen Gear
1 cup yellow lentils	1 teaspoon grated ginger	3 teaspoons ghee*	Medium pot with lid
4 cups water	½ teaspoon cumin seeds		Small frying pan
2 teaspoons chopped cilantro	1 teaspoon spice mix*		
	1 teaspoon turmeric powder		
	1 teaspoon salt		*recipe in Chapter 16

Directions

1. Soak lentils in pot of warm water for about 10 minutes. Rinse the lentils with fresh water, use your hands to move lentils until the water runs clear.
2. Add 4 cups of water and cook just over medium heat for 5 minutes.
3. As the lentils boil skim off the white foam. You may have to do this 3-4 times..
4. Reduce heat to slightly less than medium. Partially cover pot, leaving room for some steam to escape, and cook for 7-10 minutes. Add grated ginger.
5. To prepare Tarka, heat ghee in small frying pan for 15 seconds, then add cumin seeds; in about 15 seconds, add the spice mix and turmeric. Cook for another 15 seconds.
6. Add spices to the pot of lentils.
7. Take a spoonful of daal and stir it around in the tarka pan to absorb all remaining ghee and spices; stir back into the pot.
8. Garnish with cilantro and another teaspoon of ghee.

Enjoy!

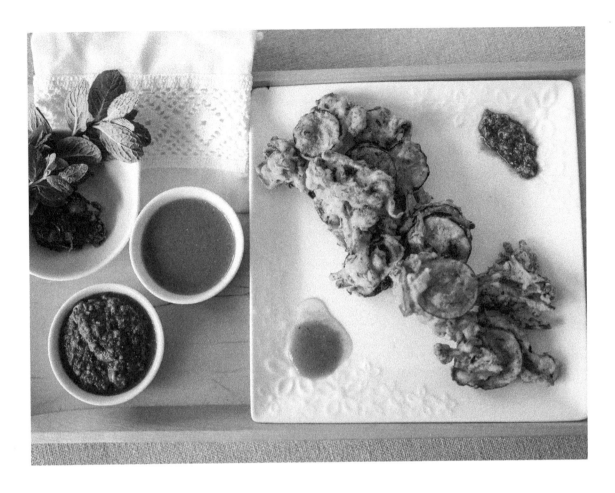

VEGETABLE FRITTERS (PAKORAS)

This is great to enjoy when you have company. It's made with chick pea flour and vegetables, all healthy stuff, and, when deep fried, it does not soak up much oil. My favorite vegetable combinations are cauliflower, potato and onions, or eggplant and onions, or spinach and onions. You can also add them all in together, or find your favorite combination. Kids love pakoras with just potatoes. It's a savory snack; serve with chai or alone as an appetizer.

- Preparation time: 25 minutes
- Serves 4-6

Main Ingredients	Herbs/Spices	Oil/Ghee	Kitchen Gear
½ zucchini cut in round slices 2 cups of cauliflower florets cut flat 1 small potato cut in thin slices 1 small onion chopped in round slices 1 cup besan (chick pea flour) 1 green chili chopped in small pieces	½ cup chopped cilantro 2 teaspoons crushed methi powder (fenugreek seed powder- optional) 1 teaspoon cumin seeds 1 teaspoon coriander seeds 1 teaspoon pomegranate seeds Dash of chili flakes Dash of black pepper 1 teaspoon salt	4 cups sunflower or safflower oil	Large bowl Deep, medium pan for frying Plate lined with paper towel Slotted serving spoon

Directions

1. Mix all chopped vegetables together in a large bowl. Add cilantro, methi powder, and all spices, including salt.

2. Set this mixture aside for 5 minutes.

3. Meanwhile, put 4 cups of oil in the pan and heat on high for 2 minutes.

4. Reduce heat to medium.

5. Add besan to the vegetables and mix well. The mix should be thick enough to coat the vegetables and you may need to add a few drops of water, a little at a time, to ensure there is enough batter.

6. Drop a tiny bit of batter into the oil: if it pops back up to the surface of the oil, it is ready.

7. Pick up the mixture with your fingers, making sure to take the vegetables and the batter together. Vegetables should be well-coated with the batter. Place in the pan – usually 5-6 pakoras will fit in a medium-size pan.

8. Use the spatula to turn pakoras to ensure they brown on all sides.

9. When pakoras are medium brown, remove with slotted serving spoon and place on paper towel-lined plate to soak up the oil.

10. Serve hot with mint and tamarind chutney.

This has been my all-time favorite snack or fun food and it's especially great for rainy and cold days. My mom would make pakoras in a big frying pan in our open kitchen. They would be picked up as soon as the spatula hit the plate and she couldn't keep up, as there were so many of us. This is undoubtedly my favorite childhood memory!

*The doctor of the future
will no longer treat the human frame
with drugs, but rather will cure
and prevent disease with nutrition.*

Thomas Edison

MORE ABOUT THE AUTHOR

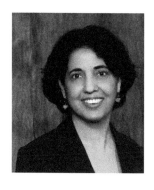

A chance Yoga class taken over 25 years ago pulled Meena Puri towards her calling of becoming a Yoga teacher and from there she found her way into the study of Ayurvedic Medicine. She has a reputation for being wise beyond her years and she is passionate about guiding people to live the purposeful lives they desire. Meena is serious—yet has a lively sense of humor—and her extensive skills allow her to transmit her profound wisdom lightly, and with ease.

Inspired by her late father, Dr. C. R. Puri, Meena's dedication to helping others is fueled by her own life's experiences, and by her conviction that we CAN heal. She has turned her own life's challenges into blessings and through her various consulting practices, she guides others to do the same. Meena credits her 22-year-old son—who she considers her biggest blessing—with teaching her the true meaning of opening her heart. In her spare time, she enjoys dancing, singing and the outdoors.

For more information on how Meena can help you derive greater health and fulfillment from your daily life, visit her website at www.ayruvedichealingcenter.com. You are invited to fill out the Initial Consultation Questionnaire on her website at https://www.ayurvedichealingcenter.com/ayurveda/initial-consulation-questionnaire/ to schedule your FREE phone consultation with her.

BIBLIOGRAPHY

- Ayurveda - The Power to Heal, Dugliss, Paul MD (2007) New World Ayurveda

- Ayurveda: A Practical Guide: The Science of Self-Healing, Lad, Dr. Vasant, (2004) Lotus Press, WI USA

- Dakshin: An Earthly Delight Cookbook: Vegetarian Cuisine from South India, Padmanabhan, Chandra, (1994) Harper Collins Publishers, San Francisco, CA

- Eat Pretty: Nutrition for Beauty Inside and Out, Hart, Jolene, (2014) Chronicle Books LLC, San Francisco

- Eat-Taste-Heal: An Ayurvedic Guidebook and Cookbook for Modern Living, Yarema, Dr. Thomas, Rhoda Daniel, and Brannigan, Chef Johnny, (2006) Five Elements Press, Kapaa, Hawai

- Enlightened Nutrition, Dugliss, Paul, MD, (2010) Perfect Paperback

- Heaven's Banquet: Vegetarian Cooking for Lifelong Health the Ayurveda Way Hospodar, Mirian Kasin, (2001) First Plume Printing, USA

- The Ayurveda Cookbook, Morningstar, Amadea and Desai, Urmila (1992) Lotus Press

- The Heartfulness Way - Heart Based Meditatiions for Spiritual Transformations, Patel Kamlesh, Pollock, Joshua. (2018) Reveal Press, Oakland CA

- You Gotta Eat: A Dietitian's Common Sense Approach to Facing Life's Health and Nutrition Challenges, Kaminski, Linda Clancy, (2011) Tanas & Associates, Farmington MI

END NOTES

1. https://www.health.harvard.edu/diet-and-weight-loss/struggling-with-emotional-eating

2. https://progressreport.cancer.gov/prevention/red.meat

3. from The Ayurveda Cookbook, Morningstar, Amadea and Desai, Urmila, Lotus Press, 1992

4. https://www.cdc.gov/foodborneburden/index.html